NOTES ON SMALL ANIMAL DERMATOLOGY

NOTES ON SMALL ANIMAL DERMATOLOGY

Judith Joyce

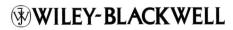
WILEY-BLACKWELL

A John Wiley & Sons, Ltd., Publication

This edition first published 2010
© 2010 Judith Joyce

Blackwell Publishing was acquired by John Wiley & Sons in February 2007.
Blackwell's publishing programme has been merged with Wiley's global Scientific,
Technical, and Medical business to form Wiley-Blackwell.

Registered office
John Wiley & Sons Ltd, The Atrium, Southern Gate, Chichester, West Sussex, PO19 8SQ,
United Kingdom

Editorial offices
9600 Garsington Road, Oxford, OX4 2DQ, United Kingdom
2121 State Avenue, Ames, Iowa 50014-8300, USA

For details of our global editorial offices, for customer services and for information about
how to apply for permission to reuse the copyright material in this book please see our
website at www.wiley.com/wiley-blackwell.

Library of Congress Cataloging-in-Publication Data

Joyce, Judith.
  Notes on small animal dermatology / Judith Joyce.
    p.; cm.
  Includes index.
  ISBN 978-1-4051-3497-2 (pbk. : alk. paper)
  1. Veterinary dermatology—Handbooks, manuals, etc. 2. Pet medicine—Handbooks, manuals,
etc. I. Title. II. Title: Small animal dermatology.
  [DNLM: 1. Skin Diseases—veterinary—Handbooks. 2. Animals, Domestic—Handbooks.
3. Skin Diseases—diagnosis—Handbooks. 4. Skin Diseases—therapy—Handbooks. SF 901 J89n
2010]
  SF901.J69 2010
  636.089'65—dc22

                                                                          2009048319

A catalogue record for this book is available from the British Library.

Set in 9/11.5 pt Sabon by MPS Limited, A Macmillan Company, Chennai, India
Printed and bound in Singapore by Fabulous Printers Pte Ltd

1 2010

Contents

SECTION 1
THE BASIC TOOLS

Chapter 1

Terminology and Glossary

Table 1.1 Terms and definitions

Term	Definition
Acanthocyte	Epidermal cell which has lost its adhesion to other cells and has become rounded, often found in sterile pustules and vesicles caused by immune-mediated disease
Acral lick dermatitis	Chronic raised erythematous lesion, usually of a distal limb, due to persistent self-trauma by licking, can develop to furunculosis
Acromelanism	Increase in hair colour at the extremities associated with lower body temperature
ACTH stimulation test	Dynamic cortisol test used in the diagnosis of hyperadrenocorticism, hypoadrenocorticism and adrenal hyperplasia like syndrome
Actinic dermatitis	Dermatitis caused by exposure to solar radiation
Adrenal hyperplasia like syndrome	Descriptive term used for a group of endocrine skin diseases causing hairloss whose pathogenesis is not totally elucidated
Allergen specific immunotherapy	Immunomodulatory treatment for atopic dermatitis using the allergens to which the patient has reacted on allergy testing
Allergy	Abnormal increased immune response to harmless foreign protein
Alopecia	Hairloss due to failure of the hair follicle
Alopecia X	See adrenal hyperplasia like syndrome
Atopic dermatitis	Skin disease caused by exposure and hypersensitivity reaction to environmental allergens
Atopy	An inherited tendency to produce IgE antibody in response to exposure to allergens
Aural haematoma	Fluid accumulation of uncertain aetiology within the cartilage affecting all or part of the pinna
Autoimmune disease	Programmed (often genetically) destruction of self-protein by the immune system
Bacterial culture	Culture of bacteria from uncontaminated samples such as pustules on a plate using growth medium
Bullous pemphigoid	Rare immune-mediated skin disease, often with poor prognosis, resembling the pemphigus group of diseases
Callus pyoderma	Chronic raised lesion with hairloss over a bony prominence subjected to friction (e.g. elbow), can develop to furunculosis
Canine/feline acne	Pustules and/or comedones on the chin with several underlying causes, similar in appearance to but differing in aetiology from human acne
Castration responsive dermatosis	See adrenal hyperplasia like syndrome
Coat brushings	Examination for surface living ectoparasites
Colour dilute follicular dysplasia	(Colour mutant alopecia) Skin condition associated with blue or fawn variants, resulting in hairloss, scaling and dermatosis, usually of dorsal head and trunk

(Contiued)

Table 1.1 (Continued)

Term	Definition
Corn	Keratin accumulation, usually of the weight bearing digital pads, often with protrusion into the dermis resulting in discomfort
Cushing's syndrome	Hyperadrenocorticism, caused by adrenal or pituitary tumour or ectopic cortisol producing tissue
Cutaneous adverse reaction to food	Skin disease caused by or exacerbated by an immunological or non-immunological reaction to ingested food
Cytology	Examination of cells and microbes by microscopy from superficial or deep skin lesions or ear canals
Deep pyoderma	Bacterial infection involving the epidermis and the dermis
Demodicosis	Dermatosis caused by multiplication of *Demodex* spp. mites within the hair follicle, usually associated with a local immune defect
Dermatophyte	Parasitic fungus, with a predilection for the hair which causes infection
Dermatophytosis	Infection caused by parasitic fungi with predilection for the hair
Dexamethasone test, high dose	Dynamic cortisol test used to differentiate pituitary and adrenal dependent hyperadrenocorticism
Dexamethasone test, low dose	Dynamic cortisol test used in the diagnosis of hyperadrenocorticism, may differentiate between pituitary and adrenal dependent cases
Diagnosis of elimination	Diagnosis which can only be reached definitively by systematically ruling out a differential list of diagnoses
Discoid lupus erythematosus	Localised immune-mediated disease, normally benign, frequently affecting the dorsal nose
Epitheliotrophic lymphoma	T lymph cell diffuse and generalised tumour of the epidermis
Erythema	Reddening of the skin due to inflammatory change
Erythema multiforme	Skin reaction pattern usually caused by immune-mediated disease, especially food or drug reaction
Exclusion diet	Diet used for food elimination trial in patients being tested for adverse cutaneous reaction to food
FCε receptor	Receptor on antigen presenting cell, specific to an antigen measured in allergy serology
Fine needle aspirate	Sample of cells ± fluid harvested from inside a lesion by suction through a 19 or 21 gauge hypodermic needle attached to a syringe
Flare factors	Extrinsic or intrinsic factors which exacerbate an existing skin disease, for example, secondary bacterial infection, hot or humid environment
Follicular dysplasia	Abnormal or incomplete structure or function of hair follicles
Folliculitis	Inflammation of the hair follicle, multifactorial including bacterial infection, ectoparasitic infestation and immune-mediated disease
Food elimination trial	Feeding an exclusion diet for the investigation of the possibility of adverse cutaneous reaction to food, usually of 3–12 weeks duration
Fungal culture	Culture of fungal elements from a plucked hair sample on a plate containing growth medium and usually a colour indicator
Furunculosis	Foreign body reaction to keratin and hair follicle components dragged into the dermis in severe and usually persistent inflammatory disease
Glabrous skin	Skin which does not normally have hair

Growth hormone responsive dermatosis	See adrenal hyperplasia like syndrome
Hair plucks	Examination of length of hair and its root grossly and by microscopically, samples harvested by epilation (see Chapter 3.3.4)
Hamartoma	Developmental raised lesion, often with change in pigmentation
Hepatocutaneous syndrome	(Superficial necrolytic dermatitis metabolic epidermal necrolysis, necrolytic migratory erythema) scaling paraneoplastic syndrome usually associated with liver and pancreatic disease
Histopathology	Microscopic examination of tissue sections by an expert
Hydrolysed diet	Diet containing nutrients of molecular weight lower than allergens used for food elimination diet, but most can be fed long term for treatment as well
Hypersensitivity	Upgraded immune response to harmless or less harmful foreign proteins
Hyperthyroidism	Disease caused by overproduction of thyroxine, usually caused by adenoma or adenocarcinoma of the thyroid gland
IDAT	Intradermal allergy testing
Idiopathic pruritus	Chronic pruritus in the dog or cat where the underlying cause cannot be identified by a thorough diagnostic workup
IgE	Reaginic antibody associated with atopic dermatitis in cats and dogs
IgE serology	Identification of antigen specific IgE (reaginic) antibody from a blood sample for diagnostic purposes in atopic dermatitis
IgG	Antibody group more generally associated with inflammatory reactions
IgG serology	Identification of antigen specific IgG antibody from a blood sample for diagnostic purposes, for example, *Sarcoptes*
Immune defect	Lack of specific part of the immune system, usually congenital, often inherited
Immune-mediated disease	Disease caused by up- or downregulation of the immune system, or abnormal response to antigens
Immunocompetence	Normally functioning immune system
Immunosuppression	Generalised reduction in function of immune system, usually due to illness or drug therapy
Impression smear	Cells, organisms and debris harvested by pressing a microscope slide onto the surface of a lesion. Usually stained for examination under high power microscope
Interdigital fistulae	Draining tracks of the tissues between the toes caused by deep pyoderma and furunculosis
Intertriginous areas	Areas of skin which rub together, sometimes resulting in maceration and secondary disease
Intertrigo	Inflammation/infection between skin folds
Juvenile cellulitis	(Puppy strangles) Immune-mediated pustular disease of puppies affecting the face usually accompanied by lymphadenopathy and systemic sig
Keratinisation defect	Defects of epidermal development usually causing greasiness and/ or scaling
Leishmaniosis	Zoonotic skin and systemic disease, prevalent in some Mediterranean countries caused by *Leishmania* spp.

(Continued)

Table 1.1 (Continued)

Term	Definition
Lentigo simplex	Normally occurring black pigment spots seen on the lips and eyelids of ginger cats
Lichenification	Thickening and texturing of the skin surface due to inflammatory change
Luminal folliculitis	Inflammation centred on the inside of the hair follicle, usually secondary to an underlying cause
Lupoid onychodystrophy	Persistent multiple nail and nail bed abnormality showing a specific reaction pattern on histopathology consistent with immune-mediated disease
Maceration	Damage to superficial tissues caused by dampness and skin folding
Macule	Discrete area of colour change not associated with skin thickening
Mass	Raised lump in the skin of any size
Metabolic epidermal necrosis	(Superficial necrolytic dermatitis hepatocutaneous syndrome, necrolytic migratory erythema), scaling paraneoplastic syndrome usually associated with liver and pancreatic disease
Mural folliculitis	Inflammation centred on the wall of the follicle, usually a primary event, often immune mediated
Muzzle	Area of the face around the nose and mouth
Myiasis	Fly strike. Blowflies lay eggs on wounds or macerated tissue. Hatched maggots then destroy further tissue
Myxomatosis	Systemic viral infection of rabbits, usually with mucocutaneous lesions, usually fatal
Necrolytic migratory erythema	(Superficial necrolytic dermatitis hepatocutaneous syndrome, metabolic epidermal necrosis), scaling paraneoplastic syndrome usually associated with liver and pancreatic disease
Nodule	Raised lump in the skin
Onychodystrophy	Disturbance in normal nail production
Papule	1–2 mm diameter discrete inflammatory lesion
Paraneoplastic syndromes	Diseases caused by primary neoplasms, with clinical signs frequently in organs distant from the site of the primary neoplasm
Paronychia	Nail bed infection
Pattern alopecia	Discrete areas of hairloss seen in particular breeds with minimal or no other skin lesions
Pemphigus	Group of immune-mediated skin diseases characterised by separation of the epidermis at different levels
Pemphigus foliaceus	Most common of the pemphigus group of immune-mediated diseases, originally considered to be autoimmune, but external trigger factors increasingly identified
Perianal adenoma	Benign tumour of the perianal glands, more common in males
Pituitary dwarfism	Congenital pituitary deficiency rarely seen in Yorkshire terriers, German shepherd dogs and others, causing persistence of puppy coat, among other signs
Plaque	Raised plate like lump in the skin
Plasma cell pododermatitis	Immune-mediated disease of the footpads of cats, usually with multiple involvement, resulting in swelling and ulceration

Pleomorphism	Variability of morphology of the cells of a single tissue type, can be indicator of malignancy
Pododemodicosis	Demodicosis of the feet alone or as part of generalised disease, often more challenging to treat
Pododermatitis	Inflammation of the feet
Pruritic threshold	Level of inflammation above which pruritus occurs, may be reached by single inflammatory diseases or combined additive effect of two or more
Pruritus	Itch
Psychogenic alopecia	Controversial diagnosis of elimination, where stress is thought to result in overgrooming and hairloss
Puppy strangles	(Juvenile cellulitis) Immune-mediated pustular disease of puppies affecting the face usually accompanied by lymphadenopathy and systemic signs
Pustule	Vesicle containing inflammatory cells with or without bacteria
Pyoderma	Bacterial skin infection
Pyotraumatic dermatitis	Bacterial infection secondary to physical damage to the skin
Recurrent flank alopecia	Benign alopecia, part of adrenal sex hormone imbalance syndrome, frequently seen in boxers, but occurs in other breeds
Sebaceous adenitis	Immune-mediated scaling disorder, resulting in destruction of hair follicles and associated glands, with strong breed predisposition
Seborrhoea	Old term for keratinisation defect (defect of epidermis), also used to describe the clinical sign of greasiness and scaliness
Skin biopsy	A full skin thickness sample harvested so as to preserve all surface, superficial and deep skin structures for examination by a dermatohistopathologist
Skin scrapes	Examination for superficial and deep living ectoparasites using samples harvested by scraping with a scalpel blade and microscopy (see Chapter 3.3.3)
Superficial necrolytic dermatitis	(Hepatocutaneous syndrome, metabolic epidermal necrosis, necrolytic migratory erythema), scaling paraneoplastic syndrome usually associated with liver and pancreatic disease
Superficial pyoderma	Bacterial infection restricted to the epidermis and hair follicles
Surface pyoderma	Bacterial infection restricted to the superficial layers of the epidermis
Systemic lupus erythematosus	Multisystemic immune-mediated disease, skin lesions varied and frequently non-diagnostic
Tape strips	Examination for surface living ectoparasites and microbes sticky tape applied to the skin surface (see Chapter 3.3.2)
Urticaria	Hives, red raised itchy lumps
Vasculitis	Inflammation of the blood vessels resulting in generalised inflammatory reaction which can be caused by drugs or infection
Vitiligo	Discrete patches of loss of pigmentation immune-mediated and possibly other causal factors
Washout period	Length of time for which a drug should be withdrawn before testing or assessing a response to treatment
Woods Lamp	Ultraviolet lamp of specific wavelength used as an aid in the diagnosis of *Microsporum* spp. of dermatophytosis (Figure 3.7)

Table 1.2 Histopathological terms

Acanthocytes	Keratinocytes which have become detached from their neighbours, usually in groups often found in immune-mediated disease, have more rounded appearance
Acantholysis	Loss of adhesion of cells, resulting in rounded cells (acanthocytes) clumping in bullae
Acanthosis nigricans	Rare pigmental disorder, usually of dachshunds
Adnexa	The structures associated with the hair follicle
Adnexal glands	Sebaceous glands associated with the hair follicles
Anagen effluvium	Loss of hair, the majority of which is in the anagen phase of growth
Anaplasia	Loss of differentiation of a cell type or tissue
Apoptosis	Cell death programmed by intrinsic or extrinsic factors (viruses, immune system, etc.), can be a primary event
Atrophy	Decrease in thickness of non-cornified epidermis due to reduced number of cells
Ballooning degeneration	Intracellular oedema, common non-specific inflammatory change
Calcinosis circumscripta	Calcium deposition in the skin due to localised disturbances in calcium metabolism
Calcinosis cutis	Calcium deposition in the skin probably due to raised mitochondrial calcium phosphate levels most commonly seen in hyperadrenocorticism
Catagenisation	'Catagen arrest'. Seen with endocrine disease and post-clipping alopecia. Follicle development stops in catagen
Cell poor interface dermatitis	Seen in specific dermatoses such as drug eruption, lupus erythematosus and toxic epidermal necrolysis
Clefts	Common artefact but also caused by acantholysis or degeneration of basal cell, occurring in inflammatory disease
Collagen atrophy	Thin fibrils with reduced fibroblasts as occurs in endocrine disease
Collagen hyalinisation	Loss of structure of collagen in the skin
Collagenolysis	Complete loss of structure of collagen in the skin
Cutaneous amyloidosis	Deposition of amyloid in the skin usually associated with more generalised amyloidosis, especially in the Sharpei
Dyskeratosis	Abnormal keratinisation (production of cornified epithelium)
Dysplasia	Abnormal or incomplete development of a tissue
Eosinophilic granuloma complex	Usually not true granulomata but raised chronic fibroplastic, sometimes eosinophilic reactions of the dermis.
Exocytosis	Migration of inflammatory cells through the epidermis, common non-diagnostic feature of inflammation
Fibroplasia	Increased amount of fibrous tissue, usually due to inflammatory skin disease
Fibrosis	Progression from fibroplasia with increased amount of fibrous tissue in the skin, little or no inflammation present but usually the result of chronic inflammation
Flame figure	Collagen surrounded by eosinophilic material indicating collagen degeneration as in eosinophilic granuloma complex and insect bites, etc.

Flame follicles	Tricholemmal keratinisation, seen in endocrine and developmental disorders
Follicular dysplasia	Incomplete or malformed hair follicles
Follicular hypertrophy	Occurs in chronic inflammation
Follicular plugging	Plugging of the hair follicle opening with keratin, common in many diseases, characteristic of some endocrine disorders
Folliculitis	Inflammation of the hair follicle, many different causes, often described by histopathologist
Furunculosis	Foreign body reaction to keratin and hair follicle components within the dermis, frequent sequel to deep pyoderma
Granuloma	Mixed and complex diffuse or nodular inflammatory reaction
Haemangiectasia	Dilation of the dermal blood vessels
Hamartoma	Mass which is a proliferation of normal or embryonic cells
Hydropic degeneration	Intracellular oedema, common non-specific inflammatory change
Hyperkeratosis	Increased thickness of cornified epithelium, found with hyperplastic epidermis in inflammatory skin conditions
Hyperpigmentation	Increased melanin deposition in the epidermis, may be primary, but common secondary to chronic inflammation
Hyperplasia	Increased thickness of non-cornified epidermis due to increased number of cells
Hypokeratosis	Reduced thickness of cornified epithelium
Hypopigmentation	Decreased melanin deposition in the epidermis
Hypoplasia	Decreased thickness of non-cornified epidermis due to reduced number of cells
Impetigo	Pustules affecting the glabrous (sparsely haired) skin of young dogs, follicles not involved
Interface dermatitis	Inflammation of the dermo-epidermal junction
Interstitial	Scattered throughout the epidermis/dermis
Interstitial dermatitis	Inflammatory cell infiltration between collagen bundles seen in a number of hypersensitivity and ectoparasite reactions
Karyolysis	Disappearance of nucleus
Karyorrhexis	Nuclear fragmentation
Keratinocyte	The living structural cell of the epidermis
Lentigo	Macule of hyperpigmentation, for example, acquired lentigo simplex of the eyelid and lips of the ginger cat
Lichenoid	Linear reaction running along or parallel to the basement membrane, usually inflammatory seen in a number of immune-mediated and other diseases
Lichenoid interface dermatitis	More 'active' inflammatory reaction of the dermo-epidermal junction seen in drug eruptions and a number of immune-mediated diseases
Luminal folliculitis	Inflammation directed at the lumen of the hair follicle
Lymphangectasia	Dilation of the dermal lymph vessels
Metaplasia	Development of cells of an abnormal type for the tissue in which they are found
Microabscess and pustules	Cavities filled with fluid and cells, the type being indicative of a diagnosis or underlying cause

(Contiuned)

Table 1.2   (Continued)

Mucinosis	Deposition of mucin in the dermis, normal in the Sharpei, seen in many inflammatory and other dermatoses including hypothyroidism
Mural folliculitis	Inflammation directed at the dermis and epidermis of the hair follicle
Necrolysis	Separation of tissue due to cell death
Necrosis	Changes seen in the cell after death
Nests	Discrete groups of cells in the dermis or epidermis, for example, lymphocytes
Nevus	Developmental defect in the skin
Orthokeratotic hyperkeratosis	Thickening of the stratum corneum with normal morphology
Panniculitis	Inflammation of the subcutaneous fat
Pansteatitis	Alteration to subcutaneous and abdominal fat due to vitamin E and essential fatty acid imbalance
Papillomatosis	Projection of dermal papillae above the skin surface, resulting in roughening of the surface, seen in inflammatory and neoplastic skin conditions
Parakeratotic hyperkeratosis	Thickening of the stratum corneum with nucleation of keratinocytes persisting, characteristic of but not diagnostic for zinc responsive dermatosis
Perivascular dermatitis	Inflammation centred on the dermal blood vessels, non-specific finding in hypersensitivity dermatitis
Pigmentary incontinence	Melanin granules free within the dermis, usually due to damage to the basement membrane zone
Pyknosis	Shrinking of nucleus
Pyogranuloma	Granuloma (mixed and complex diffuse or nodular inflammatory reaction) containing large numbers of neutrophils, for example, furunculosis
Sclerosis	End stage of fibrosis, with scar formation
Spongiosis	Intercellular oedema, common non-specific inflammatory change
Subcorneal pustule	Pustule either sterile or bacterial lying deep to the stratum corneum, occurs in a number of inflammatory and immune-mediated conditions
Subepidermal vacuolar alteration	Localised areas of separation at or below the basement membrane, occur in immune-mediated disease but common artefact
Telangiectasia	Dilation of the dermal blood vessels
Telogen effluvium	Loss of hair which has been arrested in the telogen phase due to stress, endocrine disease, etc.
Telogenisation	High proportion of hair follicles in telogen due to stress, endocrine disease, etc.
Tricholemmal keratinisation	'Flame follicles' seen in endocrine and developmental disorders
Vacuolar degeneration	Intracellular oedema, common non-specific inflammatory change
Vasculitis	Presence of inflammatory cells in and around the blood vessels, often caused by drug reactions and infection
Vesicles and bullae	Cavities filled with fluid but few cells

Chapter 2
Lesions

Some of these have been defined in Chapter 1.

The skin has a restricted number of ways of demonstrating pathology.

The appearance of the skin often depends more on the species and breed affected than the cause of the skin condition.

Clinical signs and lesions are not the same as a diagnosis and may often be unhelpful in making a diagnosis.

Acral lick lesion (Figure 2.1) Raised granulomatous or deep pyoderma/furunculosis lesion often over a leg joint due to excess licking of unaddressed/unidentified underlying dermatosis, or occasionally orthopaedic disease.

Acute moist dermatitis (Figures 2.2 and 2.3) Type of surface pyoderma characterised by acute onset (often hours) with rapid spreading from edges of lesion. Often painful and bleeding. Underlying cause often not identified but may be due to insect bite. Common in Golden and Labrador Retrievers and Rottweilers, especially on the lateral face.

Alopecia Primary lesion resulting from failure of hair follicle function, for example, endocrine alopecia in hyperadrenocorticism, leading to loss of hair.

Calcinosis cutis (Figure 2.4) Calcium deposition within the skin. May occur secondary to metabolic changes such as in hyperadrenocorticism, in which case lesions can be large and secondarily infected. Also occurs secondary to local tissue damage and foreign body invasion.

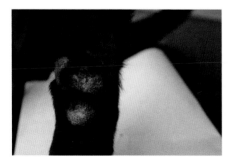

Figure 2.1 Acral lick lesion in a Labrador Retriever.

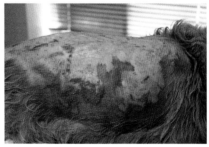

Figure 2.2 Large acute moist dermatitis lesion.

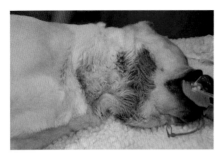

Figure 2.3 Acute moist dermatitis lesion on the face of a Labrador Retriever.

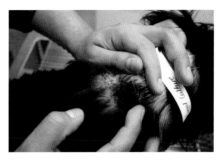

Figure 2.4 Calcinosis cutis lesion in canine hyperadrenocorticism.

Callus Abnormal thickening often associated with hairloss, lichenification, hyperpigmentation, hyperkeratosis, fissuring and occasionally secondary pyoderma, usually over a bony prominence.

Colour dilution (Figure 2.5) Genetic trait for dilution of coat colour, most commonly black becoming blue, but can be brown becoming fawn. Predisposes to follicular dysplasia.

Comedone (Figure 2.6) Keratin and sebum plug forming in hair follicle, variable in size and number. May occur spontaneously or in endocrine alopecias, primary lesion of feline acne.

Crust (Figure 2.7) Accumulation of dried exudates and 'scab' formation. May include red blood cells, inflammatory cells, serum, keratin, etc.

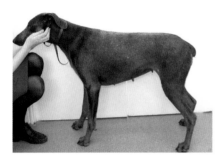

Figure 2.5 Colour dilution in a Dobermann.

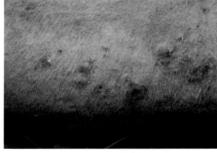

Figure 2.6 Multiple comedone formation in a Greyhound.

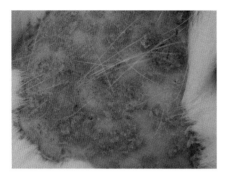 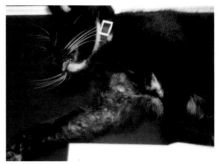

Figure 2.7 Crusting lesions on ventrum of cat. **Figure 2.8** Eosinophilic plaque.

Eosinophilic plaque (Figure 2.8) Most common lesion of the eosinophilic granuloma complex. This is a near circular raised lesion commonly produced by chronic over-grooming in cats. It is not always eosinophilic, but is a discrete thickened erythematous lesion, often close to circular. Common site is the dorsal neck or preauricular area.

Excoriation (Figure 2.9) Superficial damage to the epidermis, though may be widespread or localised, often caused by self-trauma. Does not extend to the dermis.

Epidermal collarette (Figure 2.10) Lesion remaining after a pustule bursts or resolves. Erythematous ring often raised with scaling. May be very variable in size and number. Often seen in the presence of pustules and papules.

Erythema (Figure 2.11) Early inflammatory change, persists in chronic inflammation but usually peripheral to hyperpigmentation and lichenification if present.

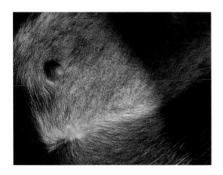 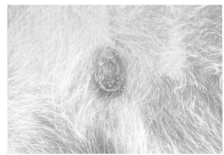

Figure 2.9 Mild erythema and excoriation. **Figure 2.10** Epidermal collarette from pustule.

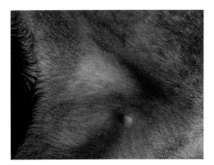

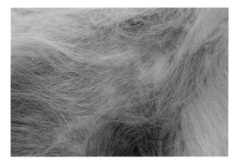

Figure 2.11 Erythema.   **Figure 2.12** Erythema multiforme.

Erythema multiforme (Figure 2.12) Unusual reaction pattern, often associated with immune-mediated disease, such as drug eruption. Often no underlying cause identified.

Feline symmetrical alopecia (Figure 2.13) Usually due to overgrooming, can be ventral or dorsal or both, not necessarily symmetrical and is not a true alopecia. Most common cause is inflammatory skin disease, usually fleas.

Fissure Split, in hyperkeratotic area, such as footpad, nasal planum and callus.

Fistulae and draining tracks (Figure 2.14) Deep lesions with tracks from the dermis or deeper. One or small numbers may be associated with foreign bodies. Multiple lesions may be indicative of deep pyoderma/furunculosis.

Furunculosis (Figure 2.15) Foreign body reaction to keratin dragged from epidermis into dermis in folliculitis and deep pyoderma.

Gingival hyperplasia (Figure 2.16) Overgrowth of gums over teeth, common in older boxers and collies. Also seen as a side-effect of cyclosporin therapy.

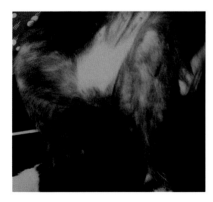

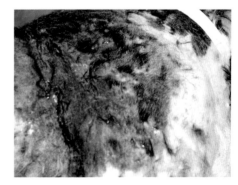

Figure 2.13 Feline symmetrical alopecia.   **Figure 2.14** Fistulae and draining tracks.

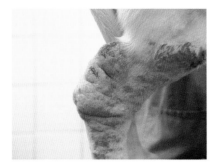

Figure 2.15 Deep pyoderma/furunculosis.

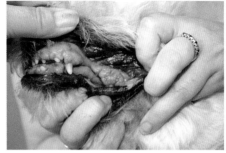

Figure 2.16 Gingival hyperplasia associated with cyclosporin therapy.

Granuloma Chronic raised or nodular inflammatory lesion identified at histopathology, may be associated with microbial infection.

Hairloss Secondary lesion resulting from many causes, often scratching, licking or biting in inflammatory skin conditions.

Hyperpigmentation (Figure 2.17) Darkening of skin may occur secondary to chronic inflammation but also occurs in other conditions.

Hygroma (Figure 2.18) Swelling over bony prominence, most frequently elbow, due to joint associated bursa filling with fluid following knocks and friction.

Intertriginous dermatitis (Figure 2.19) Surface pyoderma secondary to friction and maceration of tissues, usually in skin folds or other friction areas, for example, perineum, groin.

Lentigo Hyperpigmented macule, frequently seen as black spots on the eyelid or lip of ginger cats.

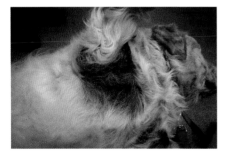

Figure 2.17 Hyperpigmentation secondary to inflammation.

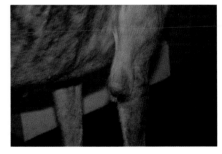

Figure 2.18 Hygroma on the elbow of a Greyhound.

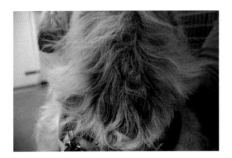

Figure 2.19 Intertriginous pyoderma of neck folds.

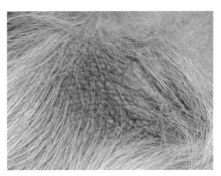

Figure 2.20 Early lichenification and erythema.

Lichenification (Figure 2.20) Cross-hatched appearance of skin and uneven thickening in response to chronic inflammation.

Linear granuloma. Lesion of the eosinophilic granuloma complex. This is a linear lesion, usually of the caudal thigh, commonly caused by chronic overgrooming in cats. It is erythematous but not always eosinophilic.

Loss of elasticity of skin (Figure 2.21) Often seen in hyperadrenocorticism in cats and dogs.

Loss of pigmentation (Figure 2.22) Loss of colour of skin, hair or mucous membranes, especially of extremities (nose, footpads, lips) though can also occur in any area, can be a sign of immune-mediated or neoplastic disease, but also occurs in scarring.

Macule Flat discrete area of change in pigmentation, not palpable.

Miliary dermatitis (Figure 2.23) Multiple 1–2 mm crusting popular lesions often associated with hairloss and broken hairs. Often dorsal lumbar region but can cover

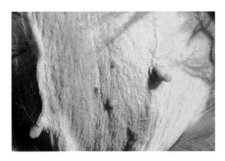

Figure 2.21 Loss of elasticity of the skin.

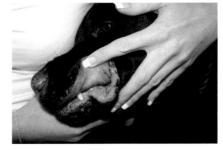

Figure 2.22 Loss of pigmentation of the lips and nasal planum in vitiligo.

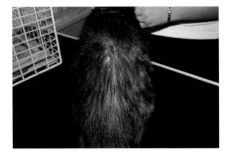

Figure 2.23 Dorsal miliary dermatitis due to flea bite reaction.

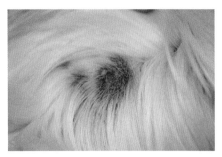

Figure 2.24 Nodular lesion.

whole dorsum, head, neck, ears, tail, and can extend down the legs and ventrally. Most common cause is primary inflammatory skin disease, usually fleas.

Nodule (Figure 2.24) Raised firm lesion, may be inflammatory, hyperplastic or neoplastic. May vary in size, colour, number and character. May be discrete or coalescing, blind or fistulating.

Papule (Figure 2.25) Raised erythematous lesion often associated with inflammation, usually 1–2 mm diameter and difficult to distinguish on gross examination from a pustule.

Pododermatitis (Figure 2.26) Inflammation of the feet, may be localised or part of a more generalised condition, often characterised mainly by saliva staining of the feet, but may also be erythematous or ulcerative, or cause lameness or secondary pyoderma with fistulae and draining tracts.

Pustule (Figure 2.27) Raised lesion containing neutrophils. Can be indicative of pyoderma in which case lesion contains bacteria and toxic neutrophils, or inflammation

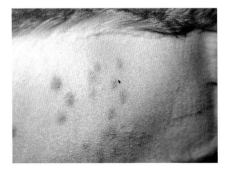

Figure 2.25 Papular reaction to flea bite.

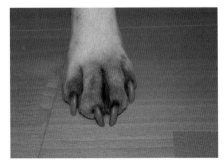

Figure 2.26 Pododermatitis.

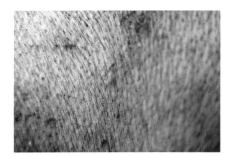

Figure 2.27 Pustule.

in which case sterile and filled with healthy looking neutrophils normally (see cytology, Chapter 3).

Rodent ulcer Name borrowed misleadingly from neoplastic lesion in man. Ulcerative mass usually on the upper lip, can be central or to either side, usually caused by over-grooming, can be useful in detection of pruritus in cats.

Scale Excess keratin shedding from the skin.

Skin thinning (Figure 2.28) Often seen with hyperadrenocorticism, cutaneous blood vessels become very pronounced.

Telangiectasis (Figure 2.29) Bleeding from cutaneous blood vessels resulting in redden-ing of the skin which is not blanched by pressure as distinct from inflammatory ery-thema. This figure shows a particularly severe case but may result in very small macules no greater than 1–2 mm diameter.

Tongue granuloma Mass on the dorsal proximal tongue, usually caused by overgroom-ing, can be useful in detection of pruritus in cats.

Ulcer Deep excoriation exposing the dermis.

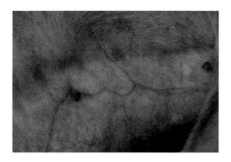

Figure 2.28 Skin thinning in hyperadrenocorticism.

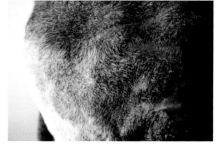

Figure 2.29 Idiopathic telangiectasis on the
shoulder of a cross-breed.

Vesicle Blister.

Wheal Response to acute inflammatory incident, leading to a swelling of short duration, often associated with erythema and pruritus and generalised swelling as in cutaneous anaphylaxis (Figure 2.30), often multiple as in hives (Figure 2.31). The diagnostic response to intradermal allergy testing.

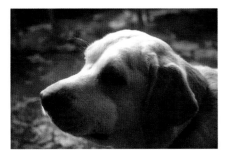 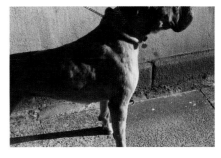

Figure 2.30 Cutaneous anaphylaxis in a Labrador.

Figure 2.31 Hives in a Boxer.

Chapter 3

Investigation and Diagnosis

This chapter is intended to help the practitioner get the most out of the case presented to them on a regular basis.

More specific diagnostic testing is included here.

A limited number of diagnostic aids are key to the diagnostic workup of most skin disease.

- Avoid the temptation to reach for empirical treatment
- Most chronic dermatoses require a definitive diagnosis for successful treatment
- It is rare for a dermatosis to be diagnosed on the basis of its presenting clinical signs
- Most diagnoses are reached by a process of elimination, so no steps should be missed

3.1 HISTORY

Necessary in all cases where the definitive diagnosis is not evident on clinical examination, for example:
- Flea bite dermatitis where live fleas visible
- Otocariasis where live *Otodectes cynotis* or *Psoroptes cuniculi* visible

Abbreviated histories and clinical examinations are adequate in acute cases where resolution is likely, for example:
- First occurrence acute moist dermatitis
- First occurrence cutaneous anaphylactic reaction
- First occurrence juvenile pyoderma
- Dermatoses where the definitive cause is demonstrated
  - Ectoparasitic disease
  - Dermatophytosis
  - Cutaneous masses

Full history and clinical examination should always be carried out in chronic, recurrent or non-responsive cases.

Form a set pattern to avoid missing important information.

Figure 3.1 is an example which can be adapted for use.
- Review regularly in persistent cases
- Beware leading questions

Breed predispositions to skin disease can be helpful in making a diagnosis, although care should be taken not to overinterpret these. Table 3.1 shows some common breeds and diseases which are considered to be common in them. There is little hard evidence to back up these clinical impressions.

3.2 CLINICAL EXAMINATION

- Full clinical examination
- Thorough examination of all areas of skin
- Always follow the same routine to avoid missing important information
- **Figure 3.2 is an example which can be adapted for use**
- Examine and record all lesions (Chapter 2)
- Record all findings
- Make an action plan

Table 3.1 Common predispositions to common diseases in common breeds

Breed	Condition
Labrador Retriever	Atopic dermatitis
	Aural haematoma
	Acute moist dermatitis
	Immune-mediated disease
Golden Retriever	Atopic dermatitis
	Acute moist dermatitis
Bull Terriers	Atopic dermatitis
	Demodicosis
	Deep pyoderma/furunculosis
Cocker Spaniel	Keratinisation defects
	Demodicosis
	Hypothyroidism
	Immune-mediated disease
Boxer	Atopic dermatitis
	Mast cell tumour
	Recurrent flank alopecia
	Hyperadrenocorticism
	Hypothyroidism
Collies	Immune-mediated disease
	Atopic dermatitis
Scottish/Cairn Terriers	Hyperadrenocorticism
West Highland White Terriers	Atopic dermatitis
	Keratinisation defects
	Demodicosis
German Shepherd Dog	Hypersensitivity dermatitis
	Deep pyoderma/furunculosis
Sharpei	Atopic dermatitis
	Demodicosis
	Hypothyroidism

HISTORY FORM

Owner's complaint

GENERAL HISTORY

Environment and lifestyle

Breed	Sex		Age
Date wormed	Date vaccinated		Neutered/Entire
Age acquired		General diet	
Other dogs	Other animals		Owners affected
Other pet contact	Wildlife/livestock contact		Travel history

Previous medical history (excluding skin diseases)

Condition	Dates	Treatments given	Response

Current Health

General Demeanour	Exercise Tolerance
Appetite Normal / Poor / Excessive / Increasing	Thirst Normal / Poor / Excessive / Increasing
Weight Thin / Fair / Good / Fat / Obese	Decreasing / Increasing / Stable
GI signs	Respiratory signs
Cardiovascular signs	Musculoskeletal signs
Neurological signs	Other

Tests performed

Test	Result

DERMATOLOGICAL HISTORY

General dermatological history

Age at onset	First signs
Severity of condition 1 2 3 4 5	Intermittent / Persistent
Improving/Stable/Fluctuating/Worsening	

Response to treatments, diets, supplements
0 = none, 2 = 20% 3 = 50%, 4 = 80%, 5 = 100%

Treatment	Names	Dates	% response	Duration of action
Drugs				
Diets				
Supplements				
Ectoparasiticides				
Other				

Owner patient score
0 = absent, 1 = mild 2 = moderate 3 = severe

	At onset	Current	Previous	Comments, triggers and spread
Itch				
Hairloss				
Smell				
Total area affected				
Spots				
Scaling and crusting				
Face				
Legs and feet				
Dorsum				
Ventrum				
Ears				

Environmental history

General Rural / Coastal / Urban / Suburban	
Daytime Inside / Outside / Car Free access / Restricted (give area)	
Nighttime Inside / Outside Upstairs / Downstairs Own bed / Owner's bed	
Bedding	**Cleaning of bedding**
Other	

Figure 3.1 History form.

CLINICAL EXAMINATION

General Examination

Eyes, ears, nose, mouth	Musculoskeletal system
Cardiovascular/Respiratory systems	GI system
Neurological signs	Other observations e.g. lymphadenopathy

Dermatological Examination

Hairloss 0 1 2 3	Erythema 0 1 2 3
Hyperpigmentation 0 1 2 3	Thickening and lichenification 0 1 2 3
Scale 0 1 2 3	Excoriation 0 1 2 3
Greasiness 0 1 2 3	Sweating 0 1 2 3

Description of lesions (see Chapter 2)

Nodules, plaques and masses	Macules/Papules/Pustules/Vesicles
Change in pigmentation	

Areas affected

Face 0 1 2 3	Ears 0 1 2 3
Periorbital skin 0 1 2 3	Axillae and groin 0 1 2 3
Feet 0 1 2 3	Legs 0 1 2 3
Dorsum 0 1 2 3	Ventrum 0 1 2 3

Areas spared

Brief summary

Action plan

Figure 3.2 Clinical examination form.

3.3 EXAMINATION FOR ECTOPARASITES

Illustrations of the common ectoparasites are shown in Figures 3.3–3.18.

The reaction patterns commonly seen with these diseases are described in Chapter 10.

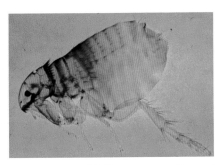

Figure 3.3 Adult flea (courtesy of Merial Animal Health).

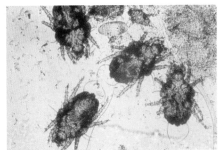

Figure 3.4 Adult *Cheyletiella* and an egg (courtesy of Merial Animal Health).

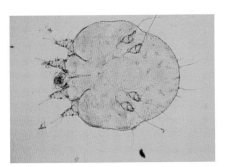

Figure 3.5 Adult Sarcoptes spp. (courtesy of Merial Animal Health).

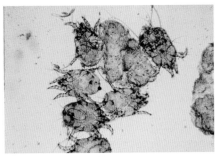

Figure 3.6 *Otodectes cynotis*, ear mites (courtesy of Merial Animal Health).

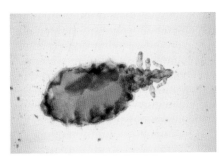

Figure 3.7 Dog louse, *Linognathus setosus* (courtesy of Merial Animal Health).

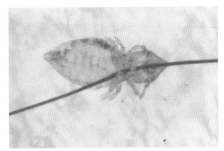

Figure 3.8 Cat louse, *Felicola subrostrata* (courtesy of Merial Animal Health).

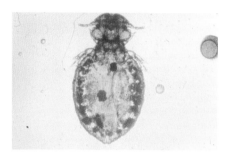

Figure 3.9 Dog louse, *Trichodectes canis* (courtesy of Merial Animal Health).

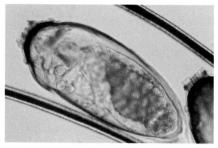

Figure 3.10 Louse egg (nit) (courtesy of Merial Animal Health).

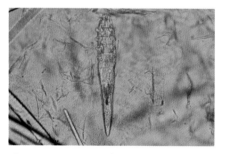

Figure 3.11 *Demodex canis* (courtesy of Merial Animal Health).

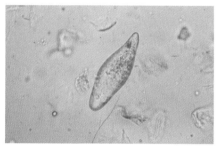

Figure 3.12 *Demodex* egg (courtesy of Merial Animal Health).

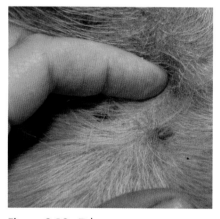

Figure 3.13 Tick.

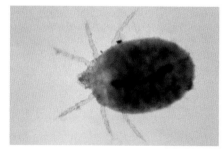

Figure 3.14 *Neotrombicula autumnalis* adult (courtesy of Merial Animal Health).

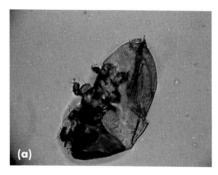 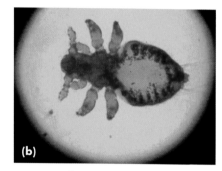

Figure 3.15 (a) Rabbit fur mite. (b) *Polyplax serrata,* mouse louse.

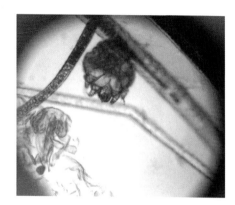

Figure 3.16 *Trixacarus caviae.*

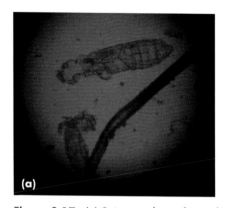 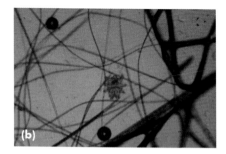

Figure 3.17 (a) Guinea pig louse. (b) *Myobia* sp.

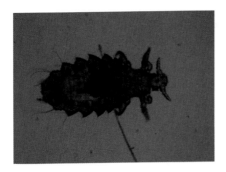

Figure 3.18 *Polyplax spinatus*, rat louse.

3.3.1 COAT BRUSHINGS

Indications
- All skin patients on first examination
- All patients presented with scaling

Coat brushings should be performed as part of a regular review of all patients undergoing treatment for chronic skin conditions.

Procedure
- Stand pet on or over large (A3) sheet of white paper
- Vigorously scratch or flea comb patient for 1 minute
- Observe paper for dark specks, light specks and movement
- Dampen dark specks with cotton wool
- Collect brushings onto microscope slide
- Examine by microscopy in liquid paraffin, low power, under cover slip

Interpretation
- Direct observation; movement may be due to presence of *Otodectes*, *Psoroptes*, *Cheyletiella* spp. (white); *Neotrombicula* spp., *Dermanyssus*, etc. (red/orange); lice.
- Wet dark specks with damp cotton wool to demonstrate the presence of flea faeces – flea faeces smudges red/brown (Figure 3.19). All samples negative on direct observation should be examined by microscopy for presence of parasites and flea faeces (Figure 3.20).
- Small amounts of flea faeces are often missed on direct observation.
- Care – various debris and pollen grains may resemble parasites and eggs.

3.3.2 TAPE STRIPS OF HAIR COAT

Indications
- Scaling dermatoses
- Suspicion of superficial ectoparasites other than fleas

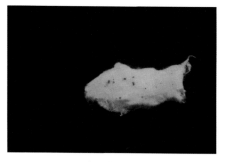

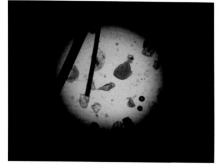

Figure 3.19 Flea faeces on damp cotton wool.

Figure 3.20 Flea faeces under microscope.

Procedure
- Scissor clip small area of hair if long haired, leaving at least ½–1″ of hair
- **Do not use clippers**
- Apply sticky side of length of transparent adhesive tape to skin surface
- Strip off tape from skin
- Stick tape to microscope slide, excluding air from underside
- Examine by microscopy, low power

Interpretation
- Presence of surface living ectoparasites, *Cheyletiella* spp. and other fur mites; lice, *Otodectes* and *Psoroptes* spp.
- Possibility of detecting non-parasitic mites or parasites from other species

3.3.3 SKIN SCRAPES

Indications
- All patients where fleas are not seen
- All patients which do not respond to a single course of treatment
- Superficial scrapes should be performed where *Sarcoptes* spp., *Notoedres* spp., *Cnemodicoptes* spp. and other superficial parasites are suspected
- Deep scrapes should be performed where *Demodex* spp. are suspected

Skin scrapes should be performed as part of a regular review of patients under treatment for chronic skin conditions.

Procedure
- Select representative area
- Choose leading edge of lesions and most recent lesions
- Scissor clip hair over affected area if necessary
- No other skin preparation should be done
- Apply liquid paraffin to affected skin
- **Superficial scrapes:** Scrape surface and crusts onto scalpel blade over about 1 cm of affected skin
- **Deep scrapes:** Scrape 1 cm × 1 cm area until capillary ooze occurs

- Transfer material to microscope slide
- Transfer large quantities of material to several microscope slides and spread
- Ensure scrapings cover slide in a thin film
- Make several slides if a lot of material
- Apply liquid paraffin
- Examine by microscopy, low power with cover slip

Interpretation
Do not rule out the presence of any ectoparasite on skin scrape.
- Presence of ectoparasites
- Scrapes of feet and chronic lesions may not reveal *Demodex*
- Multiple scrapes and examination of crusts necessary to detect *Sarcoptes* spp. still may prove inconclusive
- Superficial mites and lice may also be found
- Examination of hairs may reveal mite eggs and dermatophyte spores
- May reveal hair shaft abnormalities

A single mite, dead or alive, or its eggs is a significant finding.

3.3.4   HAIR PLUCKS

Indications
- All skin disease in cats which does not respond to flea control
- All skin disease in cats where pruritus is suspected
- Suspected dermatophytosis
- Suspected demodicosis
- Other ectoparasitic disease (less sensitive than scrapings, brushings)
- Hairloss and alopecia
- Suspected follicular defects
- Hair shaft breakage or abnormality
- Suspected endocrine disease

Procedure
- Select representative area
- No clipping or skin preparation should be done
- Pluck from recent lesions and leading edge of lesions
- Use sterile Spencer Wells forceps or similar
- Transfer to microscope slide, cover with liquid paraffin and cover slip
- Examine initially under low power

Interpretation
- Fur mites, *Cheyletiella* spp. and lice and their eggs may be demonstrated
- *Demodex* mites may be seen
- Broken hair ends indicate chewing, dermatophytosis and hair shaft abnormalities
- Follicular casts indicate keratinisation defects
- Scale attached to the hair may indicate a scaling dermatosis
- Damaged hair shafts and the presence of spores indicate dermatophytosis

3.3.5 IgG SEROLOGY

Indications
- Suspected scabies
- Undiagnosed chronic pruritic dermatoses
- Non-responsive or recurrent pruritic dermatoses

Procedure
- Submit serum sample to external laboratory

Interpretation
- Over 90% specificity
- Over 90% sensitivity

3.3.6 THERAPEUTIC TRIAL WITH ECTOPARASITICIDES

Definitive diagnosis by the methods above is preferable, but there are a number of effective broad spectrum ectoparasiticides.

As none treat all ectoparasites effectively, these should only be used following coat brushings, and superficial and deep skin scrapings to attempt to identify parasitic problems.

3.4 CYTOLOGY

Used for the examination of cells and microbes from surface, superficial or deep lesions.

Scope – surface, ears, nodules, pustules, vesicles and bullae.

Indications
- Presence or suspicion of scale, inflammatory or pigmentary change, pustules, vesicles or bullae on the skin
- Presence or suspicion of excess or altered cerumen or inflammatory change in the ears
- Pruritus or otitis
- Suspicion of altered flora on skin surface

3.4.1 SURFACE CYTOLOGY

Indications
- Ulcer, sore excoriation
- Raised mass
- Nodules

Procedure
- Select a lesional area with little hair on it
- Scissor clip the area if necessary
- No skin preparation should be done
- Rock a microscope slide back and forth over the lesion
- Leave to air-dry thoroughly
- Stain with Wright's, Giemsa or 3-step quick staining process
- Examine under high power oil immersion
- Tape strips for *Malassezia*
  - Stick on cellophane sticky tape and strip off.
  - Stick one end to each end of microscope slide, leaving a free area in the middle. Air-dry, stain as above and examine under high power oil immersion.

Interpretation
- Yeasts, bacteria and dermatophytes may be demonstrated
- For yeasts and bacteria presence of 5–10 organisms per high power field likely to be clinically significant
- Some neoplastic lesions such as suspected mast cell tumour may be diagnosed
- Some fungal granulomas may be diagnosed

3.4.2 EXAMINATION OF CERUMEN

Procedure
Take samples before any cleaning or treatment has taken place.
- Take a sample of cerumen with sterile forceps
- Add 1 drop liquid paraffin and cover with coverslip
- Examine under microscope on low power
- Using a plain bacteriological swab take a second sample and smear onto microscope slide
- Leave to air-dry thoroughly
- Stain with Wright's, Giemsa or 3-step quick staining process
- Examine under high power oil immersion

Interpretation
- *Otodectes* spp., *Demodex* spp., *Psoroptes* spp., *Sarcoptes* spp. may be seen
- The presence of *Demodex* spp. in the ear canals should alert the clinician to the possibility of systemic immunosuppressive disease, especially in the absence of other skin signs
- Parasites or their eggs, if seen, are clinically significant
- Debris, e.g. foreign body fragments, is significant
- Epithelial cells, erythrocytes and inflammatory cells are significant
- Yeasts and bacteria are found in moderate numbers in normal ears
- Twenty or more yeasts or bacteria per high power field are likely to be clinically significant (Figure 3.21 shows a normal number of *Malassezia* organisms in cerumen)

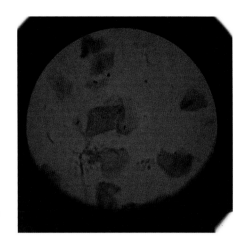

Figure 3.21 Small numbers of *Malassezia* in a cerumen sample.

3.4.3 PUSTULE, VESICLE AND BULLA CYTOLOGY

Indications
- Presence of intact pustules, vesicles and bullae which may yield diagnostic information
- Useful for differentiating sterile pustules from bacterial pustules

Procedure
- Select a large intact pustule
- Prick with 19 or 21 gauge needle
- Apply microscope slide to contents and surface of pustule, avoiding contamination from surrounding tissues
- Spread contents over slide, avoiding contamination
- Take 2–3 samples if possible
- Leave to air-dry thoroughly
- Stain 1 sample with Wright's, Giemsa or 3-step quick staining process
- Stain 1 sample with Gram stain
- Examine both under high power oil immersion

Interpretation
- Presence of bacteria and toxic neutrophils indicate pyoderma
- Absence of bacteria and healthy neutrophils indicate inflammatory process
- Acanthocytes suggest immune-mediated change
  - Figure 7.3 shows a sterile pustule. Well preserved neutrophils, no bacteria, acanthocytes
  - Figure 7.4 shows a bacterial pustule. Mature multilobulated neutrophils and intracellular bacteria
- The presence of *Demodex* is clinically significant where skin scrapes have not been diagnostic.

3.4.4 FINE NEEDLE ASPIRATE OF RAISED LESIONS

Indications
- Any firm raised mass
- Nodules
- 'Minor' lesions before considering excision biopsy
- Useful first step diagnostic procedure in some lesions which would be demanding to excise

Procedure
- Attach 21 gauge needle to 5 ml syringe
- Penetrate centre of lesion
- Apply suction to the syringe, then withdraw with suction still applied
- Remove needle from syringe, fill syringe with air then reattach
- Squirt contents onto slide
- Make multiple samples if possible
- Stain 1 sample with Wright's, Giemsa or 3-step quick staining process
- Stain 1 sample with Gram stain
- Examine under high power oil immersion

Interpretation
- Some neoplastic masses may be diagnosed, e.g. lipoma, mast cell tumour
- Some fungal and bacterial granulomas may be diagnosed
- False negatives are common; biopsy should always follow inconclusive samples
- Staging of neoplastic lesions not possible
- Submission to external laboratory will increase yield of diagnostic information
- Sensitive to operator error

3.5 SKIN BIOPSIES

3.5.1 INDICATIONS

- Nodular diseases
- Chronic non-responsive dermatosis
- The presence of alopecia, papules or pustules and scale or crust
- Skin disease with lesions characteristic for specific diseases, e.g.
  - Cutaneous masses
  - Epitheliotrophic lymphoma
  - Sebaceous adenitis
  - *Malassezia* dermatitis
  - Necrolytic migratory erythema
  - Immune-mediated disease
- Unusual presentations
- Suspected demodicosis where lesions are chronic or restricted to the feet and skin scrapes are negative
- Confirmation of diagnosis made on clinical or other diagnostic grounds
- Evaluation of secondary flare factors such as bacteria and yeast infections

- Skin disease presenting with alopecia
- Suspected hair follicle dysplasias
- Making diagnoses missed using the normal tests. Although not reliable in identifying *Sarcoptes* infection the mite in the section in Figure 3.22 was found on histopathology, despite failure to diagnose scabies on skin scrapes.

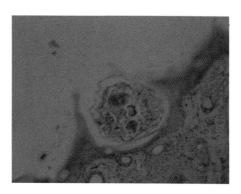

Figure 3.22 Section through sarcoptid mite in histological section (courtesy of Trevor Whitbread, Abbey Veterinary Services).

3.5.2 PROCEDURE

Many drugs, especially antipruritic agents, may alter histopathological patterns seen. Washout periods for drugs before dermatological testing are shown in Table 3.2.

The presence of severe secondary complications such as pyoderma and *Malassezia* dermatitis may obscure the primary lesions. In these cases pre-treatment for these conditions may be desirable.

- Prepare equipment
  - Labelled formalin filled universal container
  - New sterile 6–8 mm biopsy punch
  - Sterile kit comprising rat toothed forceps, scissors, needle holders, swabs
  - Piece of card for orientation of biopsies
  - Biro for marking orientation of samples
  - Monofilament nylon or staples for suturing punch holes
- Scissor clip hairy areas, avoiding skin contact
- No skin preparation should be done. Much of the important information is in the superficial layers and pustules will be damaged by contact
- Select fresh lesions with minimal secondary change
- Choose representative areas
- Do not try to include normal skin; you may miss the primary lesion
- Avoid ears noses and feet if you can (they bleed a lot)
- Don't compromise sampling when selecting the easiest areas to biopsy
- Put samples into formalin immediately to avoid loss and tissue damage
- Fill out laboratory submission form completely
- History, including treatments. and differential diagnosis are vital in interpretation
- Health and safety requirements should be followed when handling formalin
- Pack and post according to pathological specimen requirements
- Send to a dermatohistopathologist

Investigation and Diagnosis

Table 3.2 Washout periods before dermatological tests

Drug	Scrapes and brushings	Woods lamp and fungal culture	Cytology	Blood tests (see below for specific instructions)	Biopsies	Intradermal allergy tests
Shampoos	2 weeks	2 weeks	1 week	None	2 weeks	4 days
Flea treatments	6 weeks	None	None	None	None	None
Glucocorticoids	None	None	None	1 week	3 weeks	1 week off per 1 month on
Cyclosporin	None	None	None	1 week	3 weeks	1 week off per 1 month duration*
Phytopica	None	None	None	None	None	Not known
Topical steroids	1 week	2 weeks	2 weeks	None	3 weeks	None
Antihistamines	None	None	None	None	1 week	1 week
Antibiotics	None	None	1 week	None (except blood culture)	2 weeks*	None
NSAIDs	None	None	None	None	1 week	1 week

*Times are arbitrary in some cases and not always achievable.
Food elimination trial is a very demanding test and has to be discussed on a case-by-case basis.

3.5.3 INTERPRETATION

There is no such thing as a negative histopathology. As long as the sample is representative the pathologist will be able to give useful information which adds to the case information gathered.

- A non-representative sample will harvest minimal useful or even contradictory information
- A definitive diagnosis may not always be reached
- The presence of significant numbers of eosinophils in an inflammatory infiltrate is suggestive of, but not diagnostic for, ectoparasitic disease
- The presence of bacteria and *Malassezia* indicates flare factors to be controlled
- Unexpected findings allow diagnoses to be reached, e.g. the presence of ectoparasites, dermatophytes
- An unusual or difficult diagnosis is less likely to be missed
- A diagnosis should not be ruled out on the basis of a histopathology report alone – your sample may not be representative or lesions may be poorly preserved

3.5.4 READING A HISTOPATHOLOGY REPORT

A general practitioner without specialist training cannot interpret a histopathology report, but it is not necessary to do so. The following is intended to assist in getting as much out of a histopathology report as possible.

When reading a histopathology report it is important to bear the following in mind:

1 The dermatohistopathologist will only know as much of the history and clinical signs of the disease as you have given him.
2 While expert in their area, they have not seen the patient.
3 The histopathologist can only tell you what they see. The sample and its handling are all important.
4 A histopathologist will only commit to writing definite facts and opinions based on them. They may be able to discuss the case further with you verbally and interactively.

The histopathology report is divided into three sections: description, comment and diagnosis. It is tempting for the practitioner to read only the diagnosis section, but valuable information can be gained with some understanding of the other two sections.

The description may include:

- A macroscopic description of the biopsy
- A description of the changes comprising the primary lesion where a definitive diagnosis is made
- A description of the keratinised layer, epidermis and dermis
- A description of the cells seen in the biopsy and their differences from the normal where applicable
- A description of the hair follicles and adnexal structures and their differences from the normal
- The presence of micro-organisms and ectoparasites
- A description of inflammatory changes where present, including the nature of the cell infiltrate

Some descriptive histopathological terms are listed in Table 1.2. This list will not make you a dermatohistopathologist, but it should enable you to discuss cases with one.

The comment may include:

- A comparison of the four tissue samples
- A summary of the changes which are suggestive of a diagnosis
- Conditions named in the differential list for which there is no evidence
- Comments on the presence of secondary flare factors, such as yeasts and bacteria
- Comments on hair follicle and sebaceous gland activity
- Comments on the presence and nature of hyperkeratosis
- A thought process which does not reveal a diagnosis but invites discussion
- Suggestions for further investigations which may be indicated
- Comments on the limitations imposed by samples, sampling or information provided

Diagnosis

- Definitive diagnosis where one has been made
- Prognosis where a definitive diagnosis has been made
- Differential diagnosis where a definitive diagnosis has not been made
- Comment on the severity and significance of complicating factors such as secondary bacterial infection
- Sometimes treatment suggestions are made

3.6 FUNGAL EXAMINATION

Indications
- All feline dermatoses where fleas have not been demonstrated to be the cause
- All feline dermatoses in breeding or showing colonies
- Whenever two or more in contact animals share a dermatosis
- Newly acquired young animals
- Newly acquired animals from rescue centres
- All chronic, recurrent or non-responsive dermatoses
- All small mammal dermatoses
- Scaling dermatoses
- Alopecic dermatoses

3.6.1 DIRECT MICROSCOPY

Procedure
- Where there are no discrete lesions the pet should be brushed all over for 1 minute onto a large sheet of paper (Mackenzie brush technique)
- Alternatively, a hair pluck is taken from the edge of a recent lesion
- Hair pluck may be guided by Woods Lamp examination
- The sample is transferred to a microscope slide, covered with liquid paraffin and a coverslip; alternatively stain with polychromatic methylene blue
- Spores may be seen on the hairs

Interpretation
- Technically demanding, hence false positives and false negatives occur
- Presence of spores indicates dermatophytosis
- Fungal hyphae also seen invading hairs
- Use an external laboratory unless experienced and for a definitive diagnosis

3.6.2 WOODS LAMP EXAMINATION (FIGURE 3.23)

Procedure
- Use in a completely darkened room
- Some species of dermatophyte fluoresce under ultraviolet light
- Good quality Woods Lamp required of adequate power and narrow waveband
- Switch lamp on 10 minutes prior to use to ensure consistent wavelength
- Scan entire pet for at least 10 minutes
- Some hairs may take up to 5 minutes to fluoresce

Interpretation
- Woods Lamp examination cannot be used to rule out a diagnosis of dermatophytosis.
- Positive results are indicated by a bright apple green fluorescence (Figure 11.6).
- False positives caused by:
  ○ Other substances fluorescing
  ○ Overinterpretation of fluorescence

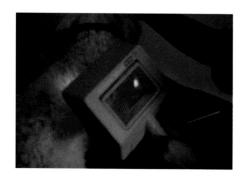

Figure 3.23 Woods Lamp examination.

- False negatives caused by:
  - Non-fluorescent species of ringworm. *Trichophyton* dermatophytes do not fluoresce and only 60% of *Microsporum* spp. fluoresce
  - Wrong wavelength of inadequate power
  - Inadequate warm-up time for lamp
  - Inadequately darkened room
  - Inadequate scanning of patient
  - Topical treatments masking lesions
  - Absence of fresh lesions

3.6.3 FUNGAL CULTURE

Procedure
- Where there are no discrete lesions the pet should be brushed all over for 1 minute onto a large sheet of paper (Mackenzie brush technique)
- Alternatively, a hair pluck is taken from the fresh edges of a recent lesion
- Hair pluck may be guided by Woods Lamp examination
- In-house fungal culture can be done using colour changing dermatophyte test media (Figure 3.24)
- Culture may take 4–6 weeks at room temperature
- Most colour changes occur within 2 weeks
- Colour change should be visible before colony growth
- Culture plates should be examined daily for colour change followed by colony growth

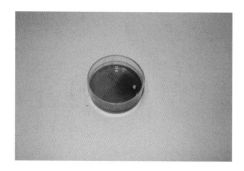

Figure 3.24 Positive *Trichophyton* culture on in-house dermatophyte medium.

Interpretation
- Rapid colour change indicates preferred protein metabolism of parasitic species of fungi
- Acidic breakdown products of protein metabolism result in colour change to red. This occurs more slowly with non-parasitic species as they metabolise carbohydrates first, but colour changes are eventually seen with saprophytic species
- Colour change in 10–14 days followed by white fluffy culture growth in 2–6 weeks is indicative of dermatophytosis
- False negatives and positives can be caused by contamination of the plates
- False negatives can result from early reading of results
- False positives can result from late reading of results wzen both colour change and colony growth have occurred
- False positives can result from growth of non-parasitic fungi

In challenging cases and where species identification is required, submission to an external laboratory is mandatory.

Human infection may be useful in the diagnosis of especially feline ringworm (Figure 3.25) as most species of dermatophyte are zoonotic. However, human medical practitioners are apt to overdiagnose dermatophytosis contracted from pets in their patients. Conversely, if dermatophytosis is suspected clients should be warned as dermatophytosis can be serous in young children and immune-suppressed or diabetic individuals.

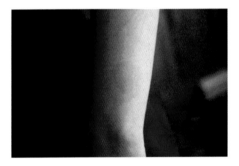

Figure 3.25 Ringworm lesion on the arm of a veterinary nurse.

3.7 EXAMINATIONS FOR BACTERIA AND YEASTS

3.7.1 CYTOLOGY

See above.

Interpretation
- Surface cytology indicated in suspected *Malassezia* overgrowth, more than 5 organisms per high power field
- Pustule cytology indicated in pyoderma
- Ceruminal cytology useful in otitis externa

3.7.2   BACTERIAL CULTURE

- Little useful information can be obtained from swabs taken from the surface of the skin or open lesions. Bacterial samples should be submitted to a professional laboratory for accurate culture and identification.

Interpretation
- Swabs taken from intact pustules can be helpful in the choice of antibiotic to be used, but care should be taken to identify any persisting underlying causes
- Culture from cerumen may be helpful in the choice of antibiotic to be used in otitis externa, but the underlying cause must always be addressed

3.8   ALLERGY TESTING

3.8.1   INVESTIGATION OF SUSPECTED ADVERSE CUTANEOUS REACTION TO FOOD

Indications
- First step in allergy testing
- Dermatoses with concurrent dietary intolerances

Procedure
1   The gold standard test for adverse reaction to food remains the 12 week home-cooked diet using a novel protein source and a novel carbohydrate source with no additives.
2   Hydrolysed diets of restricted molecular weights of less than 10,000 Da may be a useful compromise solution where it is not possible to use a home-cooked diet. Lower molecular weight diets may be preferable.
3   Commercial restricted protein source diets may contain trace quantities of other proteins which may trigger an adverse food reaction resulting in failure of food trials.
4   The use of intradermal allergen testing and in vitro serological testing for specific IgG and IgE remains controversial at the time of writing.

The procedure for a food elimination trial is described in detail in Chapter 12. This should be read carefully before embarking on food elimination trials, along with the flow chart (Figure 12.2).

Patients should not be on drugs to control pruritus during the trial (see Table 3.2).

Appendix 1 is a handout for clients which can be adapted for use when conducting food elimination diets in practice.

Interpretation
- Dermatoses due to adverse cutaneous reactions to food should respond to dietary trial in 12 weeks
- Relapse should occur on provocation with other foodstuffs
- Condition should be well controlled on diet without specific allergen(s)
- Avoid confusion with feeding diets high in essential fatty acids and other cofactors for amelioration of skin conditions

3.8.2 TESTS FOR ENVIRONMENTAL ALLERGENS IN THE MANAGEMENT OF ATOPIC DERMATITIS

A diagnosis of atopic dermatitis cannot be made on the basis of these tests alone.

Allergen serology

Indications
- History and clinical signs consistent with atopic dermatitis
- Ectoparasitic disease ruled out first
- Cutaneous adverse reaction to food ruled out first where possible

Procedure
- Tests for IgE serology and FCɛ receptor serology available commercially
- Initial screen followed by expansion panels usually performed
- Can select expansion panel initially based on history and clinical signs
- Washout periods for drugs (Table 3.2)

Interpretation
- According to laboratory's guidelines and advice
- False positives and false negatives occur
- IgE scores below the laboratory threshold do not rule out allergens
- IgE scores above the laboratory threshold are strongly suggestive but not necessarily diagnostic
- Scores based on IgG levels should be viewed with caution
- Test demonstrates patient's ability to produce IgE (the reaginic antibody) to the specific allergen; it does not necessarily mean that the cause of the skin problem is due to those allergens
- Results of serological testing must be interpreted in combination with history and clinical signs
- Results of ASIT based on serology have been similar to those following IDAT

Intradermal allergy testing

Indications
- History and clinical signs consistent with atopic dermatitis
- Ectoparasitic disease ruled out first
- Cutaneous adverse reaction to food ruled out first where possible

Procedure
- Use non-antihistaminic sedation
- Opioids have been reported to alter reactions
- General anaesthesia may be necessary in cats, especially in expanded tests
- Use commercially available kits; either single or multiple allergens can be used
- Washout period for drugs (Table 3.2)
- Clip hair from a lesional area of skin on flank
- Indelibly mark areas to be injected
- Inject 0.05–0.1 ml allergens
- Measure reaction at 15 minutes and 1 hour in dogs, 5 minutes and 15 minutes in cats

Interpretation
- Considered still to be the gold standard test
- Demonstrates a skin reaction to allergens
- False negatives and false positives occur due to:
  - Poor technique
  - Irritant reactions, especially mites
  - Insufficient washout periods
  - Lack of response possibly due to 'exhaustion' towards the end of the allergy season
  - Lack of response possibly due to 'unprimed' immune system out of the allergy season
  - All positive due to generalised reaction
- Small, difficult to read reactions can occur, especially in cats

3.9 TESTS FOR ENDOCRINE DISEASE

3.9.1 HYPOTHYROIDISM

Indications
- History and clinical signs consistent with hypothyroidism
- Non-pruritic skin disease
- Hairloss with or without systemic signs
- Recurrent or persistent pyoderma
- Scaling disease

Procedure (see Table 3.3)
- Basal total T4 may be performed as screening test, but is affected by other illnesses and concomitant drug therapy, and a reliable diagnosis cannot be made by total T4 assay alone
- Diagnosis can be made on abnormal free T4 by equilibrium dialysis and TSH assay
- Dynamic tests (TRH or TSH stimulation test)

Interpretation
- Blood biochemistry and complete blood count (CBC) screening tests may include T4 and may be indicative but are not diagnostic alone (see Table 3.3)
- Beware euthyroid sick and drug suppression causes of low T4
- T4 by equilibrium dialysis combined with TSH assay is diagnostic of hypothyroidism
- TRH/TSH stimulation tests can be used in inconclusive cases

3.9.2 HYPERADRENOCORTICISM

Indications
- History and clinical signs consistent with hyperadrenocorticism (HAC)
- Non-pruritic skin disease
- Hairloss with or without systemic signs
- Recurrent or persistent pyoderma
- Scaling disease
- Poorly controlled diabetes mellitus

Table 3.3　Blood sampling in dermatological disease

	Time for test	Protocol	Sample(s) required	Special instructions
General health profile	Single sample	Haematology and biochemistry to include manual differential	EDTA Heparin Fluoride oxalate (glucose)	Steroids will affect results
Thyroid screen	Single sample	Free T4 by equilibrium dialysis	Serum	Free T4 by equilibrium dialysis is best screening test
Thyroid test	Single sample	Free T4 by equilibrium dialysis, TSH assay	Serum	
Dynamic thyroid tests TRH or TSH stimulation tests	4 hours	IV protirelin/TSH after basal sample taken, take second sample after 4 hours	2×serum	TSH is expensive TRH test is more difficult to interpret
ACTH stimulation test	1 hour	IV synacthen after basal sample taken, take second sample after 1 hour	2×serum	Less sensitive test but more forgiving of test conditions
Low and high dose dexamethasone tests	8 hours	IV 0.01 mg/kg (low dose) or 0.1 mg/kg (high dose) Dexamethasone after basal sample taken, take samples at 3 and 8 hours	3×serum	Sensitive test but very susceptible to error in practice
Endogenous ACTH assay	Single sample but transport arrangements must be made in advance	Take blood, spin and freeze serum immediately. Transport frozen	Serum	Very reliable test, contact investigating laboratory to arrange transport and avoid weekends
Adrenal hyperplasia like syndrome	1 hour	ACTH stimulation test (see above) and measurement of cortisol and oestradiol	2×serum	Contact investigating laboratory
Sarcoptes or allergen serology	Single sample	Allergen specific antibody or receptors measured	At least 3 ml serum	Steroid withdrawal similar to intradermal test for some
Coombs tests	Single sample		1×serum	Contact laboratory for interpretation
ANA	Single sample		1×EDTA	Contact laboratory for interpretation

Pre-test fasting is advisable in most cases. 12 hours before all blood samples are taken, except for some post pilling samples where treatment has to be given with food. Refer to investigating laboratories for reference ranges and submission protocols.

Procedure (see Table 3.3)
- Blood biochemistry and CBC may be helpful indicators but not diagnostic
- Basal cortisol levels, not diagnostic alone
- ACTH stimulation test
- Low and high dose dexamethasone tests
- Urinary cortisol/creatinine ratio
- Ultrasound imaging of adrenal glands
- MRI
- Contrast CT imaging
- Scintigraphy

Interpretation (see Chapter 14)
- High fasting glucose, raised liver enzymes, leucocytosis, neutrophilia and eosinopaenia all indicative
- ACTH stimulation test – high basal and/or excessive increase in cortisol after stimulation diagnostic (use reference ranges of external laboratory used)
- Low dose dexamethasone suppression test. Suppression at 3 and 8 hours diagnostic for HAC
- High dose dexamethasone test
  - Suppression at 3 hours and lack of suppression at 8 hours diagnostic for pituitary dependent HAC (PDHAC)
  - Suppression at 3 and 8 hours suggestive of adrenal dependent HAC (ADHAC)
- High endogenous ACTH indicative of PDHAC, low exogenous ACTH indicative of ADHAC
- Ultrasound imaging useful in the diagnosis of ADHAC but technically demanding

3.9.3 OTHER ENDOCRINE ALOPECIAS

Indications
- Alopecias, not suggestive of thyroid or adrenal disease

Procedure (SHAP profile)
- ACTH stimulation test combined with oestradiol assay (see Table 3.3)
- Submit to external laboratory

Interpretation
- Consult external laboratory for reference ranges
- Tentative diagnosis on values outside normal ranges
- Normal ranges do not eliminate diagnosis, but consider seasonal flank alopecia and reconsider hair follicle dysplasias on normal values

SECTION 2
PROBLEM-ORIENTATED APPROACH

Chapter 4
The Pruritic Patient

4.1 CAUSES OF PRURITUS

- There is evidence that pruritus pathways are separate from pain pathways so that pruritus is not pain to a lesser degree
- Pain can block out pruritus
- Pruritus can block out pain

4.1.1 MAJOR DERMATOLOGICAL CAUSES

- Ectoparasites
- Hypersensitivity dermatitis
- Pyoderma
- Other skin infections
- Secondary complications of non-pruritic skin disease, e.g. pyoderma secondary to hypothyroidism, calcinosis cutis

4.1.2 NEUROLOGICAL CAUSES

- Inherited sensory neuropathies
  - English Pointers
  - Dachshunds
- Acquired sensory neuropathy
  - Canine ganglioradiculitis
  - Aujesky's disease
  - Peripheral nerve tumours
  - Paraneoplastic peripheral neuropathy
- Cutaneous manifestations of CNS disease
  - Syringohydromelia associated with Arnold Chiari Syndrome in Cavalier Spaniels
- Psychomotor or partial complex seizures

4.1.3 BEHAVIOURAL CAUSES

- Displacement behaviour
- Tail chasing (Bull Terriers)
- Flank sucking (Dobermanns)
- Pruritus associated with CNS tumours reported in humans
- Myoclonus of distemper may resemble pruritus and cause skin lesions

Pruritus due to dermatological causes will be described in more detail. Neurological and behavioural causes can usually only be investigated further once the dermatological causes have been ruled out.

4.2 THE PRURITIC DOG

Table 4.1 shows the primary and secondary lesions commonly associated with pruritus in the dog.

- More obvious in the dog than the cat
- Main signs are scratching, nibbling at the body and foot chewing
- Head-shaking, face-rubbing and 'scooting' may also be present

Figure 4.1 outlines the management of the dog with generalised pruritus. The numbers in the text refer to the numbers on the figure.

Localised pruritus may also be caused by:
- Demodicosis
- Dermatophytosis
- Neoplasia resulting in the release of inflammatory cytokines
  ○ Mast cell tumour
  ○ Langerhans cell tumour
- Contact irritant
- Insect bites and stings
- Anal sac disease

Localised pruritus should be investigated for these common causes before considering more generalised diseases where localised self-trauma may occur due to accessibility and habituation.

Table 4.1 Lesions commonly associated with pruritic dermatological disease in the dog

Primary lesions	Secondary lesions
Papule	Acral lick lesion
Pustule	Acute moist dermatitis
Nodule	Crust
Vesicle	Excoriation
Bulla	Epidermal collarette
Wheal	Erythema
	Fistulae and draining tracks
	Granuloma
	Intertriginous dermatitis
	Lichenification
	Scale
	Hyperpigmentation

These lesions are described in Chapter 2.

The Pruritic Patient

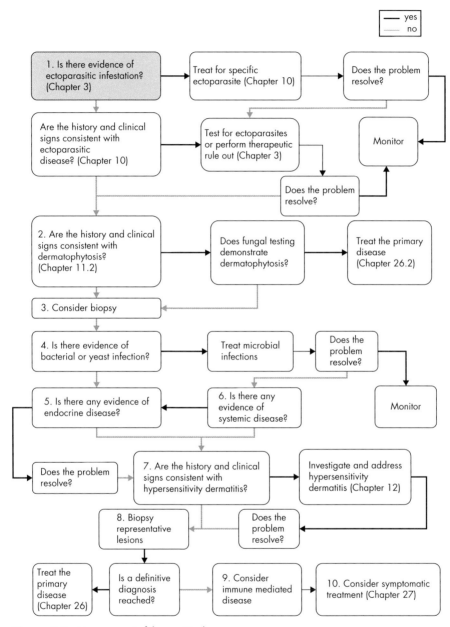

Figure 4.1 Management of the pruritic dog.

4.2.1 ECTOPARASITES

Ectoparasites are the most common cause of pruritus in the dog. The first step in the investigation of persistent or recurrent pruritus is a thorough investigation for the presence of ectoparasites.

It is recognised that patients suffering from atopic dermatitis are more likely to demonstrate hypersensitivity reactions to flea bites than dogs with normal skin, so long-term aggressive ectoparasite control is important.

Scabies can mimic the clinical signs of atopic dermatitis and can also be challenging to demonstrate on skin scrapes. IgG serology or a therapeutic trial for *Sarcoptes* spp. should be performed at the start of an investigation for hypersensitivity dermatitis.

4.2.2 DERMATOPHYTOSIS

Dermatophytosis is relatively uncommon in adult pet dogs in temperate and cold climates. Many dermatologists perform fungal culture as part of their screening pruritic cases. However, fungal testing should always be carried out in:

• Young dogs
• Dogs from refuges
• Non-responsive cases
• Localised pruritus, especially when accompanied by scaling

4.2.3 BIOPSY MAY BE CONSIDERED AT THIS STAGE

Although histopathological changes are not pathognomonic in many cases of pruritus, biopsy at an early stage may be useful:

• To rule out conditions which may resemble hypersensitivity dermatitis (see Chapter 4.2.7)
• To establish the presence of microbial infections
• To establish the degree of secondary change

4.2.4 BACTERIAL AND YEAST INFECTIONS

Bacterial and yeast infections are a common cause of pruritus in dogs.

Most bacterial and yeast infections are secondary to an initiating cause.

If bacteria and yeast infections do not respond to appropriate treatment (**see Chapters 26 and 27**), **an underlying cause should be identified and addressed.**

Common causes include:

• Immaturity
• Ectoparasitic disease
• Inflammatory skin disease
• Immunosuppressive skin disease
• Endocrinopathy

4.2.5 ENDOCRINE DISEASE

Endocrine skin disease does not generally cause pruritus.

However, pruritus can be caused commonly by:

- Demodicosis in hyperadrenocorticism
- Dermatophytosis in hypothyroidism or hyperadrenocorticism
- Secondary microbial disease in endocrinopathy
- Calcinosis cutis in hyperadrenocorticism

4.2.6 SYSTEMIC DISEASE

Immunosuppressive disease may result in secondary pruritic microbial disease.

Some systemic diseases commonly demonstrate skin lesions which may result in pruritus.

- Paraneoplastic syndromes
- Zinc responsive dermatosis

4.2.7 HYPERSENSITIVITY DERMATITIS (CHAPTER 12)

Hypersensitivity dermatitis is at times the most common cause of pruritus.

Parasitic hypersensitivity to fleas, *Sarcoptes* spp. or *Otodectes* spp. should be ruled out first by taking coat brushings, skin scrapes and cerumen samples and where necessary IgG serology for *Sarcoptes* spp. and therapeutic trial.

Adverse cutaneous reaction to food should be investigated by elimination diet.

If clinical signs and history are consistent with atopic dermatitis, allergy testing should be carried out if allergen specific immunotherapy is to be considered.

Where bacterial, yeast or fungal infections are a significant feature, hypersensitivity to bacteria, fungi or *Malassezia* spp. should be considered.

4.2.8 BIOPSY REPRESENTATIVE LESIONS

See Chapter 3 for indications and procedure for taking histopathological specimens.

If a definitive diagnosis has not been reached, biopsies should be taken to rule out conditions which resemble hypersensitivity dermatitis such as:

- Immune-mediated disease (see Chapter 13)
- Diseases of the pilosebaceous unit (see Chapter 15)
- Epitheliotrophic lymphoma which can present as a scaling erythematous condition in the early stages (see Chapter 16)

4.2.9 IMMUNE-MEDIATED DISEASE (SEE CHAPTER 13)

Immune-mediated disease cannot be ruled out on histopathological examination.

The history, clinical signs and any trigger factors should be reviewed at this stage.

The Pruritic Patient

The Pruritic Patient

4.2.10   IDIOPATHIC PRURITUS

Idiopathic pruritus is a diagnosis of elimination which may be considered at this stage after a careful review of the history, clinical signs and diagnostic tests.

Long-term symptomatic control is normally the only option in these cases (see Chapter 27.1).

4.3   THE MORE MATURE PATIENT

The preceding differential diagnoses should still be considered in these patients, but additionally there is an increased incidence of the following conditions.

4.3.1   ENDOCRINOPATHIES (CHAPTER 14)

Although not primarily pruritic, these conditions frequently result in pyoderma, scaling or other lesions which can cause pruritus.

- Diabetes mellitus
- Hypothyroidism
- Hyperadrenocorticism

4.3.2   METABOLIC DISEASES (CHAPTER 17)

- Hepatic disease – hepatocutaneous syndrome
- Renal disease

4.3.3   NEOPLASIA (CHAPTER 16)

- Primary neoplasia
  - Epitheliotrophic lymphoma
  - Mast cell tumours
- Secondary neoplasia
- Paraneoplastic syndromes (Chapter 16)

4.4   THE PRURITIC CAT

The investigation and management of feline skin conditions present quite different challenges from those encountered in treating dermatoses in the dog.
1   Cats are very secretive and do not demonstrate the presence of pruritus or discomfort in an obvious way.
2   Macroscopic lesions are frequently limited and not pathognomonic for or indicative of one particular disease.

3   The types of lesions associated with feline dermatoses are very limited.
4   Patient and owner compliance for oral treatments is frequently poor.
5   Patient and owner compliance for therapeutic trials, e.g. food elimination diet, ectoparasite rule outs is frequently poor.
6   Patient and owner compliance for topical treatments is frequently poor and therefore useful adjunctive therapy is often limited.

Some dermatoses, such as plasma cell pododermatitis, will present with a typical clinical appearance and occasionally the underlying cause of an ectoparasite infestation will be found readily, but most cases present a significant diagnostic challenge.

4.4.1   RECOGNITION OF PRURITUS IN THE CAT

Evidence of pruritus is usually related to the presence of overgrooming.

Overgrooming is frequently not evident to the owner.

The evidence below will usually convince both the clinician and the owner of the presence of a pruritic skin condition.
1   Hairloss, symmetrical or non-symmetrical
2   Miliary dermatitis
3   Presence of lesions due to self-trauma
4   Evidence of ectoparasites
5   Presence of scale, crust, papules, etc.
6   Microscopic examination of hair for broken ends
7   Furball vomiting or obstipation
8   Fur attached to tongue papillae
9   Presence of oral or lip 'granulomas'
10   Faecal examination for hair, ectoparasites, etc.

The absence of scale, crust, papules, ectoparasites does not rule out pruritic skin disease in cats as they may remove all evidence during overgrooming.

4.4.2   LESION PATTERNS IN CATS

Lesion patterns in cats can be valuable in establishing the presence of pruritic skin disease.

Cats react to pruritic dermatoses in three main ways:
1   Miliary dermatitis
2   Feline symmetrical alopecia
3   Eosinophilic granuloma complex

It is important to remember that these three reaction patterns do not represent a diagnosis but merely a description of lesions which may be caused by a number of pruritic conditions. They may be present in isolation or in combination and, although some patterns are more commonly associated with certain diagnoses, it is possible for any dermatosis to produce any of these lesions.

Miliary dermatitis (Figure 2.23)
Table 4.2 lists the common differential diagnoses for cats presenting with miliary dermatitis.

Table 4.2 Differential diagnosis of miliary dermatitis/symmetrical alopecia in cats (common diagnoses in bold)

Ectoparasitic disease	**Flea bite dermatitis**
Fungal diseases	**Dermatophytosis**
	Malassezia dermatitis
Viral diseases	(FeLV and FIV related dermatoses)
Other parasitic skin diseases	***Otodectes cynotis* acariasis**
	Louse infestation
	Neotrombicula autumnalis
	Cheyletiellosis
	Sarcoptes scabiei infestation
	(*Notoedres cati* infestation)
	(Fur mites)
	Demodicosis
	(Accidental infestations from prey)
Allergic skin diseases	**Flea hypersensitivity dermatitis**
	Adverse reaction to food
	Atopic dermatitis
	Contact dermatitis
Immune-mediated disease	**Pemphigus foliaceus**
	Other types of pemphigus
	Drug eruption
	(Bullous pemphigoid)
	(SLE)
	(DLE)
	Erythema multiforme
	(Vasculitis)
	Alopecia areata
Endocrine and metabolic disorders	**Prednisolone side-effects**
	Hyperthyroidism
	Diabetic dermatosis
	HAC
	Paraneoplastic syndromes
	(Oestrogen responsive dermatosis)
Other acquired alopecias	**Telogen defluxion**
	Traction alopecia
	Topical glucocorticoid application
	(Paraneoplastic alopecia)
	Follicular dysplasia
	Pattern alopecias
Neoplasia	Epitheliotrophic lymphoma
	Secondary skin neoplasia
	Exfoliative dermatitis associated with thymoma
Keratinisation defects	Primary seborrhoeic conditions
	Secondary seborrhoeic conditions
Other	Psychogenic alopecia
	Feline hypereosinophilic syndrome

- Very common reaction pattern in early skin disease
- Not diagnostic for an underlying cause
- Easily recognised by owner
- Dorsal papular crusting lesions about 1–2 mm diameter
- Often associated with hairloss and skin thickening

Feline symmetrical alopecia (Figure 2.13)

Table 4.2 lists the common differential diagnoses for cats presenting with symmetrical alopecia.

- Not diagnostic for an underlying cause
- Usually ventral, may not be symmetrical, variable in extent
- Often goes unnoticed by owner
- Hair shortening rather than total loss may be seen
- Microscopic examination of hair plucks reveals broken and damaged hairs
- Skin biopsy often reveals little evidence of inflammatory skin disease, but normal hair follicle function is seen

For many years this lesion was thought to be evidence of hormonal skin disease in cats. Owners often still believe this to be the case as they are not aware of their cat overgrooming.

Eosinophilic granuloma complex (Figure 2.8)

Table 4.3 lists the common differential diagnoses for cats presenting with lesions of the eosinophilic granuloma complex.

These lesions are not true granulomas; they are a chronic inflammatory reaction to self-trauma, usually by a cat's rough tongue.

The underlying causes are many, but their presence is often suggestive of chronicity.

It is important to differentiate these lesions from neoplasia at an early stage.

1 **Linear granuloma:** perhaps the most common presentation. It is seen as a raised erythematous linear lesion most commonly on the caudal aspect of one or both hindlimbs.
2 **Eosinophilic plaques** are also very common and appear as raised lesions of various shapes and sizes over various parts of the body. They are often found on the trunk and dorsal neck.
3 **Indolent ulcer** (rodent ulcer). These are found on the lip margins and again are the result of excessive grooming. There may also be oral and tongue ulceration.

Facial pruritus

Table 4.4 lists the common differential diagnoses for cats presenting with facial pruritus.

Facial pruritus is a less common presentation of the eosinophilic plaque.

Table 4.3 Differential diagnosis of eosinophilic granuloma complex in cats (common diagnoses in bold)

Ectoparasitic disease	**Flea bite dermatitis**
Fungal diseases	**Dermatophytosis**
	Malassezia dermatitis
Viral diseases	(FeLV and FIV associated dermatoses)
	Feline calicivirus infection
	Feline poxvirus infection
	(Feline papillomavirus)
Other parasitic skin diseases	***Otodectes cynotis* acariasis**
	Louse infestation
	Neotrombicula autumnalis
	Cheyletiellosis
	Sarcoptes scabiei infestation
	(*Notoedres cati* infestation)
	(Fur mites)
	Demodicosis
	(Accidental infestations from prey)
Allergic skin diseases	**Flea hypersensitivity dermatitis**
	Adverse cutaneous reaction to food
	Atopic dermatitis
	Contact dermatitis
Immune-mediated disease	Other types of pemphigus
	Drug eruption
	(Bullous pemphigoid)
	Erythema multiforme
	(Vasculitis)
	(TEN)
Endocrine and metabolic disorders	Diabetic dermatosis
	HAC
	Paraneoplastic syndromes
Neoplasia	Sarcoma
	Mast cell tumours
	Squamous cell carcinoma
	Epitheliotrophic lymphoma
	Secondary skin neoplasia
Keratinisation defects	Primary seborrhoeic conditions
	Secondary seborrhoeic conditions
Other	Feline hypereosinophilic syndrome
	Idiopathic sterile granuloma
	Some nevi

The Pruritic Patient

It has been said in the past that facial lesions are more likely to be related to food hypersensitivities, but there is little evidence to support this.

Facial pruritus lesions, however, may be more challenging to manage.

Characterised by erythematous ulcerated discrete plaque-like lesions in the preauricular area, it has also been said that facial pruritus is more difficult to control than the other reaction patterns. It is characterised by erythematous, often ulcerated in

Table 4.4 Differential diagnosis of facial pruritus (common diagnoses in bold)

Ectoparasites	**Flea bite dermatitis**
Fungal Diseases	**Dermatophytosis**
	Malassezia dermatitis
Other parasitic skin diseases	***Otodectes cynotis* acariasis**
	Louse infestation
	Neotrombicula autumnalis
	Cheyletiellosis
	Sarcoptes scabiei infestation
	(*Notoedres cati* infestation)
	(Fur mites)
	Demodicosis
	(Accidental infestations from prey)
Allergic skin diseases	**Flea hypersensitivity dermatitis**
	Adverse cutaneous reaction to food
	Atopic dermatitis
	Contact dermatitis
Immune-mediated disease	**Pemphigus foliaceus**
	Other types of pemphigus
	Drug eruption
	(Bullous pemphigoid)
	(SLE)
	(DLE)
	Erythema multiforme
	(Vasculitis)
	Alopecia areata
Endocrine and metabolic disorders	Diabetic dermatosis
	HAC
	Paraneoplastic syndromes
	(Oestrogen responsive dermatosis)
Neoplasia	Sarcoma
	Mast cell tumour
	Squamous cell carcinoma
	Epitheliotrophic lymphoma
	Secondary skin neoplasia
	Exfoliative dermatitis associated with thymoma
Keratinisation defects	Primary seborrhoeic conditions
	Secondary seborrhoeic conditions
Other	Idiopathic facial dermatitis
	Feline solar dermatitis
	Idiopathic sterile granuloma
	Some nevi
	Feline hypereosinophilic syndrome

the preauricular region. There may also be a miliary dermatitis of the face and head, associated with skin thickening and folding.

The differential diagnosis for each lesion pattern is extensive.

The most common cause of pruritus in cats is fleas. It has been estimated that at some times of year 98% of cats presenting with dermatological problems have evidence of fleas.

4.4.3 PRINCIPLES OF INTERPRETING CUTANEOUS REACTION PATTERNS

1 The reaction patterns represent the ways in which feline skin can respond to inflammation.
2 No reaction pattern is indicative of a single diagnosis.
3 Any inflammatory skin disease can respond by producing any of the reaction patterns.
4 Neoplasia must be ruled out at an early stage in the presence of any raised erythematous or ulcerated lesion.
5 Only a small number of differential diagnoses are common, most are rare.

The list of differential diagnoses for the major skin reaction patterns in the cat is shown in Tables 4.2–4.4.

4.5 CLINICAL APPROACH TO THE PRURITIC CAT

Figure 4.2 outlines the management of the pruritic cat. The numbers in the text refer to the numbers on the figure.

4.5.1 TREAT ECTOPARASITE INFESTATIONS AND RULE OUT OR CONTROL FLEA BITE DERMATITIS

Flea bite dermatitis is the most common diagnosis in first opinion veterinary practice and a significant number of feline patients referred for second opinion have a definitive diagnosis of flea bite dermatitis.

Diagnosis of the presence of fleas and dermatitis due to flea bites remains surprisingly challenging, but it is imperative to rule out ectoparasite problems before moving on to the second stage of diagnostic workup.

The following steps are essential in ruling out flea bite dermatitis in the pruritic cat. Even then flea bite dermatitis remains a flare factor that should be continually addressed.
1 Careful examination of the hair coat for fleas and flea dirt
2 Gross examination of coat brushings with the owner present
3 Microscopic examination of coat brushings
4 Aggressive flea control with adulticides and insect growth regulators
5 Microscopic examination of faeces for fleas
6 Examination of coat brushings (gross and microscopic) from other animals in house
7 Microscopic examination of hair for broken ends, indicating the presence of pruritus
8 Full clinical examination of cat for evidence of overgrooming
9 Review flea control
10 Start to consider other diagnoses, but maintain flea control and monitor regularly

A cat who is grooming excessively may remove all outward evidence of flea infestation. In these cases evidence of infestation in other animals in the household may be invaluable and examination of faeces for flea body parts and hair chewed out can also help.

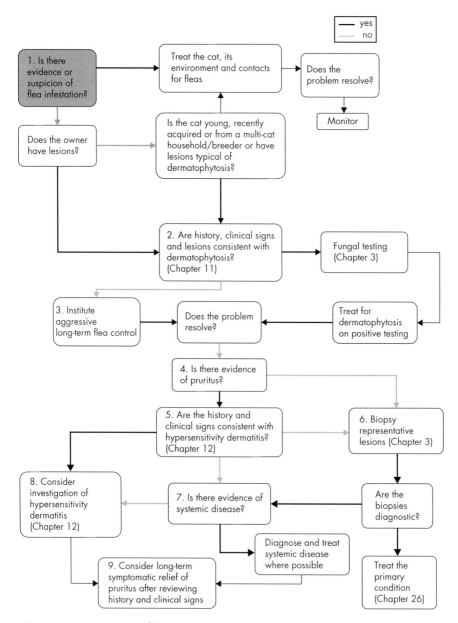

Figure 4.2 Management of the pruritic cat.

4.5.2   INVESTIGATE THE POSSIBILITY OF DERMATOPHYTOSIS

Dermatophytosis is common in colonies of cats, newly acquired kittens and in some multi-cat households. Although the truism that, if it looks like ringworm, it probably isn't, often holds, the possibility of dermatophytosis should be considered at an early stage in the investigation of all feline skin disease. Woods Lamp examination is a useful screening test, but the diagnosis cannot be ruled out without negative fungal culture. Direct microscopy for fungal spores is a procedure which, even in experienced hands, can give false negative (and positive) results. A laboratory experienced in the culture and identification of fungal organisms should be used, although in-house dermatophyte culture media can be a useful back up. Dermatophytosis may present without lesions, with or without scaling, pruritus, hairloss or erythema in a localised or more generalised form. Its zoonotic potential, especially in immunocompromised humans, should be taken seriously.

4.5.3   INSTITUTE LONG-TERM FLEA CONTROL

Flea bite dermatitis is the most common cause of feline skin disease.

Flea bite dermatitis is the most common flare factor in chronic feline skin disease.

Feline atopic dermatitis patients may be more susceptible to flea bite dermatitis.

4.5.4   ESTABLISH THE PRESENCE OF PRURITUS

Most common dermatological problems in the cat are pruritic. Cats tend not to scratch but rather groom excessively when they are pruritic and, since they are frequently secretive groomers, this may not be evident to the owner. The next step in the diagnostic workup of skin diseases in cats therefore is usually to establish the presence of pruritus and demonstrate this to the owner.

Evidence for the presence of pruritus in the cat is listed in Section 4.4.1.

4.5.5   TAKE A FULL HISTORY AND CLINICAL EXAMINATION

While most cases of skin disease in cats are caused by fleas and it is acceptable to investigate and treat for fleas and dermatophytosis before taking a full history, it is important not to miss the diagnosis in recurrent or non-responsive cases.

Full clinical histories should be taken in the following cases:

- Failure to respond to appropriate flea control
- Failure to respond permanently to an appropriate therapeutic trial
- Unusual appearance of lesions

The Pruritic Patient

- Evidence or suspicion of systemic disease
- Recurrent or persistent skin disease
- Evidence of zoonotic infection

4.5.6 SKIN BIOPSY

Skin biopsy should be undertaken in all non-responsive cases of feline skin disease where a thorough ectoparasite and dermatophyte rule out has been undertaken. The technique for taking diagnostic skin biopsies is described in Chapter 3.

It is important to take skin biopsies early in non-responsive cases where there are raised, plaque-like or ulcerative lesions to rule out the possibility of neoplasia.

4.5.7 SYSTEMIC DISEASE AS A CAUSE OF PRURITUS

Skin disease in cats can be a useful indicator of internal disease. Healthy cats are fastidious groomers and an unkempt appearance or the presence of a large number of ectoparasites, such as fleas or lice in the coat should lead the clinician to consider a diagnostic workup for systemic disease.

Several systemic diseases have been associated with dermatological disease.

- Paraneoplastic syndromes such as exfoliative disease in thymoma, superficial necrolytic dermatitis (hepatocutaneous syndrome, metabolic epidermal necrosis, necrolytic migratory erythema)
- Predisposition of cats to demodicosis and scabies (*Sarcoptes scabiei*) in the presence of immunosuppressive disease
- Hyperthyroidism and hyperadrenocorticism

It has been suggested that a dermatosis may occur in association in FIV positive cats.

4.5.8 INVESTIGATE POSSIBILITY OF HYPERSENSITIVITY DERMATITIS (SEE CHAPTER 12)

Hypersensitivity dermatitis is common in cats but is still quite poorly understood. The main types are:

- Parasitic hypersensitivity (fleas, ear mites)
- Environmental allergy (house dust mites, pollens, etc.)
- Cutaneous adverse reaction to food
- Contact dermatitis (may be causes other than hypersensitivity)
- Other more rare hypersensitivities

4.5.9 SYMPTOMATIC RELIEF OF PRURITUS (SEE CHAPTERS 26.3 AND 27.1)

Where it is not possible to establish the underlying cause of pruritus, long-term antipruritic treatment is usually required.

Long-term aggressive flea control is essential.

Regular review of the history and clinical signs to confirm the diagnosis and address flare factors is essential.

Chapter 5
The Scaling Patient

Also known as keratinisation defects and seborrhoea.

Seborrhoea is an old term fallen into disuse, useful descriptively but not diagnostically.

Mild scaling

- May be cosmetic, requiring symptomatic or no treatment
- May be precursor of more serious scaling disease
- May be harbinger of systemic disease

Primary scaling problems

- Uncommon
- The most commonly encountered conditions are listed in Table 5.1
- Often inherited, particular breeds predisposed
- Usually a diagnosis of elimination or have pathognomonic changes on histopathology
  Limited treatment options
- Long-term palliative treatments nearly always needed

Secondary scaling problems

- Much more common
- The most common causes of scaling disorders are listed in Table 5.2
- Occurs secondary to many other skin diseases
- Significant scaling a feature of some dermatoses – may aid diagnosis

Excess scaling is less frequently seen in cats as they remove scale with excessive grooming. This makes diagnosis of scaling disorders more challenging as scale, and parasites and micro-organisms that are the most common underlying causes are frequently removed by the tongue.

Figure 5.1 outlines the management of scaling conditions in the dog and cat. The numbers in the text refer to the numbers on the figure.

5.1 THE MOST COMMON CAUSE OF SCALING CONDITIONS IS PARASITES

Scaling is frequently seen in flea bite dermatitis.

Dorsal scaling and pruritus are important diagnostic features of cheyletiellosis and louse infestation.

Localised or generalised demodicosis may initially present as a mild scaling dermatosis with associated hairloss and minimal to absent pruritus.

Table 5.1   Some diseases where scaling is the primary lesion

Immune-mediated dermatoses	Sebaceous adenitis Pemphigus
Endocrinopathy	No common conditions
Diseases of the pilosebaceous unit	Colour dilution alopecia Hair follicle dysplasias Sebaceous adenitis
Neoplasia and paraneoplastic diseases	Epitheliotrophic lymphoma, superficial necrolytic dermatitis exfoliative dermatitis associated with thymoma
Nutritional diseases	Essential fatty acid deficiency Vitamin A deficiency Zinc responsive dermatosis
Localised diseases	Nasal and digital pad hyperkeratosis Ear margin dermatosis
Other	Idiopathic mural folliculitis, lichenoid dermatosis, contact irritant dermatitis
Congenital and hereditary defects	Hairless breeds of dog and cat Colour dilute alopecia Black hair follicle dysplasias Vitamin A responsive dermatosis Zinc responsive dermatosis Ichthyosis Primary keratinisation defect especially of Cocker Spaniels

Table 5.2   Skin diseases commonly resulting in secondary scaling

Cause	Examples
Ectoparasitic disease	Cheyletiellosis Louse infestation
Micro-organisms	*Malassezia* dermatitis Leishmaniosis
Hypersensitivity dermatitis	Parasitic hypersensitivity Atopic dermatitis Cutaneous adverse food reaction Contact dermatitis Other
Immune-mediated disease	Pemphigus complex especially pemphigus foliaceus, DLE, SLE, drug eruption
Endocrine and metabolic disease	Canine hypothyroidism Feline hyperthyroidism Hyperadrenocorticism Diabetes mellitus Sex hormone dermatoses, including testicular tumours, adrenal hyperplasia like syndrome Glucocorticoid administration Paraneoplastic syndromes
Localised skin diseases	Solar/actinic dermatitis Symmetrical lupoid onychodystrophy

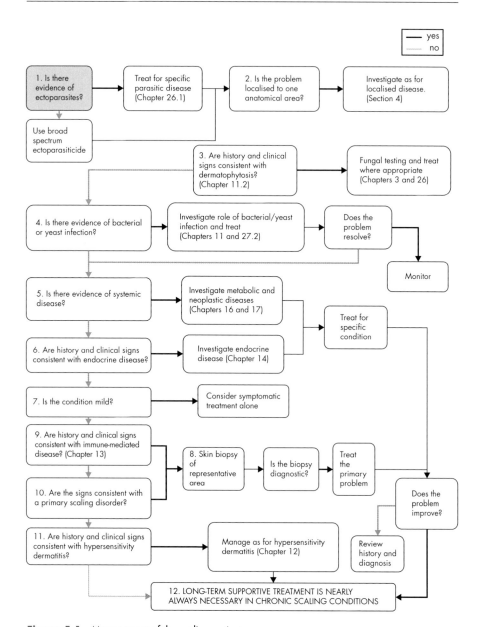

Figure 5.1 Management of the scaling patient.

The Scaling Patient

5.2 LOCALISATION OF SCALING DISORDERS

Scaling is most frequently generalised but can be localised to especially

- Nasal planum (Chapter 22)
- Digital pad (Chapter 18)
- Ear margin (Chapter 20)

Distribution of lesions is often helpful in determining the underlying cause

- Ectoparasitic disease
- Pemphigus foliaceus
- Superficial necrolytic dermatitis ('hepatocutaneous' syndrome)
- Sebaceous adenitis

5.3 DERMATOPHYTOSIS

Dermatophytosis should be considered early in the investigation of all cases of scaling, especially in cats, rabbits and rodents.

All localised scaling lesions should be screened for dermatophytosis in these patients (Chapter 3).

5.4 BACTERIAL AND YEAST INFECTIONS

Malassezia dermatitis is a common cause of scaling in the dog, cat and rabbit although there is usually an underlying disease which predisposes the pet to infection.

Bacterial pyoderma may result in scaling and should be considered, even in the absence of visible pustules. Leishmaniosis should also be considered (Chapter 11.1).

5.5 SYSTEMIC DISEASE

Systemic disease is a common cause of scaling dermatoses.

Scaling frequently precedes systemic signs:
1 If excess scaling or greasiness is seen in cats, causes of reduced grooming should be considered, for example,
    - Oral disease
    - Musculoskeletal disease
    - Obesity, usually apparent
    - Debilitating systemic disease
2 Nutritional disease. Most modern diets carry concentrated amounts of nutrients but for example, reduced protein, zinc and essential fatty acid availability can lead to scaling dermatoses (Chapter 17)
3 Metabolic disease (Chapter 17)

4 Neoplastic conditions (Chapter 16)
- Epitheliotrophic lymphoma frequently presents as a scaling dermatosis of gradual onset
- Paraneoplastic syndromes such as:
  - Superficial necrolytic dermatitis
  - Exfoliative dermatitis in thymoma
5 Endocrine dermatoses (Chapter 14)

5.6 ENDOCRINE DISEASE

Endocrine disease, especially in the early stages or in canine hypothyroidism, may present with skin signs alone.

Endocrine disease should not be ruled out until either a definitive diagnosis has been made or endocrine screening tests have been performed, especially in less pruritic scaling dermatoses.

5.7 MILD SCALING

Many scaling dermatoses are mild and mainly a cosmetic problem.

Examples include:

- Scaling following a moult or mild inflammatory reaction
- Scaling following illness or stress as in telogen defluxion
- Scale occurring secondary to the follicle dysplasias such as colour dilution alopecia

Dilute coat colour may be sufficient evidence of underlying follicle dysplasia to justify diagnosis and treatment on colour and age alone.

A minimum of coat brushings, skin scrapes and tape strips should be carried out in these cases to avoid missing treatable primary causes such as ectoparasites and *Malassezia* spp.

It is important to consider systemic causes and neoplastic of scaling dermatosis before treating conservatively or symptomatically.

Dogs with a history of foreign travel or non-responsive or systemic signs should also be investigated for leishmaniosis.

Additional essential fatty acid, zinc and vitamin E may be beneficial in these patients. These are available in commercial diets as well as dietary supplements (Chapter 27).

Topical treatment is very useful and frequently underused in scaling dermatoses (Chapter 29).

Cases which are treated conservatively should be monitored carefully for improvement. Non-responsive and recurrent cases should be investigated promptly.

5.8 BIOPSY

Biopsy should be considered in all recurrent and non-responsive scaling dermatoses or those with an unusual presentation where scaling is the most prominent clinical sign.

The technique for obtaining diagnostic skin biopsies is described in Chapter 3.

5.8.1 IN SOME CASES BIOPSY MAY BE DIAGNOSTIC

- Sebaceous adenitis
- Superficial necrolytic dermatitis
- Some cases of immune-mediated disease
- Skin neoplasia, e.g. epitheliotrophic lymphoma
- Zinc responsive dermatosis
- Hair follicle dysplasias
- Demodicosis where mites have not been found on skin scrapes
- Dermatophytosis

5.8.2 BIOPSY MAY BE SUPPORTIVE OF PROVISIONAL DIAGNOSIS

- Vitamin A responsive dermatosis
- Endocrine dermatosis
- Immune-mediated skin disease
- Zinc responsive dermatosis
- Drug eruption
- Hypersensitivity dermatitis
- Ectoparasitic disease

5.8.3 SECONDARY COMPLICATING FACTORS

The presence and extent of secondary complicating factors such as pyoderma and *Malassezia* dermatitis can be evaluated.

5.9 IMMUNE-MEDIATED DISEASE

Pemphigus foliaceus, the most common of the pemphigus group of diseases, usually presents as a scaling dermatosis. Other forms of pemphigus may also cause scaling.

Sebaceous adenitis is an immune-mediated disease of predisposed breeds which frequently presents with marked dorsal, often symmetrical scaling, with or without gross evidence of inflammation.

Investigation of immune-mediated disease is described in Chapter 13.

5.10   PRIMARY GENETIC SCALING DISORDERS

These frequently present with secondary inflammatory skin conditions, but may present without any other signs. They are diagnosed by ruling out the causes of secondary scaling disorders, supported by histopathological changes.

5.11   HYPERSENSITIVITY DERMATITIS

Scaling is a very common secondary lesion in hypersensitivity dermatitis.

Investigation of hypersensitivity dermatitis is described in Chapter 12.

Secondary *Malassezia* dermatitis will cause marked scaling and greasing.

5.12   TREATMENT OF SCALING DISORDERS

See Chapter 27.3.

Where possible the primary underlying cause should be addressed.

Long-term supportive therapy is usually necessary in scaling dermatoses other than those caused by ectoparasites.

Topical treatments and dietary supplements are often beneficial.

Secondary microbial infections are common in scaling dermatoses.

Chapter 6
The Alopecic Patient

There are two types of loss of hair coat:
1   Hairloss following damage to the hair follicle as a result of inflammation or trauma.
2   True alopecias where hairloss is the primary event due to follicular failure.

It is often difficult to differentiate these problems on history and clinical signs alone.

There are some strong breed predispositions to some alopecias and these may help in preparing a list of differential diagnoses.

Table 6.1 shows a list of the common breed predispositions.

However, it is important not to disregard the possibility of other causes of hairloss in these breeds.

Figure 6.1 outlines the management of hairloss in the dog and cat. The numbers in the text refer to the numbers on the figure.

6.1   CONGENITAL OR INHERITED HAIRLOSS

Some pets who are born without normal hair coats have been bred for a genetic trait. This is often associated with abnormalities of keratinisation which require lifelong control. Similarly, congenital hair coat defects are generally resistant to treatment and the best treatment methods are aimed at improving comfort and appearance. These conditions are relatively rare but are outlined in Chapter 15.

6.2   PATTERN ALOPECIAS

These occur in a number of breeds and are not associated with other dermatosis, for example, pinnal hairloss in the dachshund. Treatment is not usually necessary although palliation may be required if there is secondary scaling. There is an increased risk of trauma to the pinna in the absence of a protective hair coat.

6.3   TRAUMATIC HAIRLOSS

Patients will sometimes present with patchy hairloss following injury, burns (especially from exhaust pipes following road traffic accidents), abscess or pyoderma. Owners should be warned that the prognosis for hair regrowth is very variable. There is little treatment possible.

Topical applications can also result in patchy hairloss. Withdrawal of treatment may result in hair regrowth. This commonly occurs with glucocorticoids and spot or line-on ectoparasiticidal products.

Care should be taken to rule out dermatophytosis and demodicosis in these cases.

Table 6.1 Breeds commonly predisposed to primary alopecic conditions

Breed	Condition
Airedale	Non-colour linked follicular dysplasia Recurrent flank alopecia
Alaskan malamute	Adrenal hyperplasia like syndrome
American Water Spaniel	Pattern baldness
Boxer	Recurrent flank alopecia Hyperadrenocorticism Hypothyroidism
Boston Terrier	Pattern baldness
Chihuahua	Colour dilute follicular dysplasia Pattern baldness
Curly coated retrievers	Non-colour linked follicular dysplasia
Dachshund	Pattern baldness Pinnal alopecia
Doberman	Colour dilution follicular dysplasia Non-colour linked follicular dysplasia
English Bulldog	Pattern baldness
Greyhound, Whippet, Italian Greyhound	Colour dilute follicular dysplasia Pattern baldness
Irish Water Spaniel	Non-colour linked follicular dysplasia
Maltese Terrier	Traction alopecia
Manchester Terrier	Non-colour linked follicular dysplasia Pattern baldness
Miniature Pinscher	Non-colour linked follicular dysplasia
Miniature poodle	Adrenal hyperplasia like syndrome Hyperadrenocorticism
Pomeranian	Adrenal hyperplasia like syndrome
Portuguese Water dog	Non-colour linked follicular dysplasia Pattern baldness
Rhodesian ridgeback	Pattern baldness
Staffordshire Bull Terrier	Pattern baldness
Yorkshire Terrier	Traction alopecia Pinnal alopecia Hyperadrenocorticism Pituitary dwarfism

The Alopecic Patient

6.4 INFLAMMATORY HAIRLOSS

It is important, but often difficult, to differentiate alopecia where hairloss results from failure of the hair follicle and secondary hairloss which arises from damage to the hair shaft or the hair follicle. This is particularly challenging in the cat where apparently non-inflammatory hairloss due to hypersensitivity dermatitis and dermatophytosis is common. Management of inflammatory hairloss is described in Chapters 4 and 5.

The Alopecic Patient

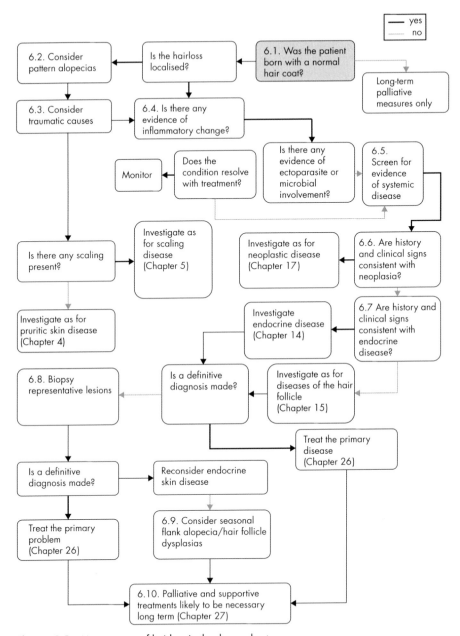

Figure 6.1 Management of hairloss in the dog and cat.

6.4.1 EVIDENCE FOR INFLAMMATORY HAIRLOSS

1 Evidence of pruritus
   • Licking, biting scratching, head-shaking
   • Evidence of fur ingestion
   • Tongue or lip lesions

2   Evidence of hair breakage on microscopic examination
3   Demonstration of ectoparasites and/or response to ectoparasiticides
4   Demonstration of dermatophytes and response to treatment
    (Application of collars to prevent licking without antipruritic therapy should be
    avoided.)
5   Bacterial and yeast cultures

6.5   SCREEN FOR ALOPECIA DUE TO SYSTEMIC DISEASE

Patients with generalised alopecia should be screened for systemic disease. Where
the history and clinical signs are consistent with endocrine or neoplastic disease,
haematological and biochemical investigation is indicated. Neoplastic, endocrine
and organic disease should be considered. Table 6.2 lists the main alterations in
haematological and biochemical parameters which may occur in commonly occurring endocrine disease. Although not diagnostic these are indications that endocrine
disease should be investigated further in the presence of a supportive history and
clinical signs.

6.6   PARANEOPLASTIC ALOPECIA

This is a rare condition but should be investigated where clinical signs and history are
consistent with neoplasia.

6.7   ENDOCRINE ALOPECIA

Causes of endocrine and non-endocrine alopecia are shown in Table 6.3.

Endocrine alopecia should be differentiated from non-endocrine causes of alopecia.
Evidence which may be helpful:

• History and clinical signs
• Presence of inflammatory change
• Lack of systemic clinical signs
• Normal haematological and biochemical parameters
• Normal results for specific endocrine blood tests
• Biopsy may be helpful
• Frequently a diagnosis of elimination

There is no single test which can definitively diagnose each condition – a diagnosis can
be reached following:

• History and clinical signs consistent with the endocrine disease
• Supportive haematological and biochemical examinations
• Basal and dynamic endocrine blood tests
• Occasionally supportive histopathology is required

Endocrine disease is described in Chapter 14.

The Alopecic Patient

Table 6.2 Changes in blood parameters in common endocrine disease

Diabetes mellitus	Hypothyroidism	Hyperadrenocorticism
Hyperglycaemia	Mild regenerative anaemia	Leucocytosis
↑ alkaline phosphatase	↑ alkaline phosphatase	Neutrophilia
↑ cholesterol	↑ cholesterol	Eosinopaenia
		Lymphopaenia
		Mild/moderate hyperglycaemia
		↑ alkaline phosphatase
		↑ cholesterol
		↑ ALT

Table 6.3 Causes of hairloss

Endocrine alopecia	Non-endocrine alopecia	Secondary hairloss
Hypothyroidism	Alopecia areata	Demodicosis
Hyperadrenocorticism	Lymphoma	Dermatophytosis
Gonadal sex hormone alopecia	Recurrent flank alopecia	Other ectoparasitic disease
Adrenal hyperplasia like syndrome	Telogen defluxion	Hypersensitivity dermatitis
Pituitary dwarfism	Traction alopecia	Staphylococcal pyoderma
	Feline paraneoplastic alopecia	Mural folliculitis
	Injection site reaction	Vasculitis
	Dermatomyositis	Scarring
	Ischaemic dermatosis	Lymphoma
	Congenital alopecia	Immune-mediated disease
	Follicular dysplasias	
	Colour dilution follicular dysplasia	
	Black hair follicular dysplasias	
	Pattern baldness	

Thorough and sometimes repeat testing after 3–6 months is often required to reach a diagnosis.

A diagnosis of endocrine disease can rarely be definitely ruled out.

6.8 BIOPSY

Histopathological changes are uncommonly specific for one endocrine disease, despite the existence of characteristic cellular changes in each disease due to secondary changes.

Supportive histopathology can help the clinician to reach a definitive diagnosis.

Some non-endocrine alopecias are frequently diagnosed by a combination of history, clinical signs and histopathological changes.

Biopsy is important to rule out paraneoplastic syndromes and neoplastic disease.

A complete review of the diagnosis and management of all alopecias should be carried out at intervals unless the disease is clinically insignificant.

6.9   NON-ENDOCRINE ALOPECIAS

It is often important to reassure the client that the condition is benign.

Repeat endocrine testing after a period of time will reveal some endocrinopathies.

Complicating skin diseases are common in endocrine skin disease:

- Demodicosis
- Pyoderma
- *Malassezia* dermatitis
- Dermatophytosis

Progression of the existing disease.

6.10   LONG-TERM PALLIATIVE TREATMENT IS USUALLY NECESSARY IN ALOPECIC SKIN CONDITIONS TO ADDRESS SECONDARY COMPLICATIONS (SEE CHAPTER 27)

Primary treatment of the diagnosed problem may not result in total resolution of the clinical signs – scaling and secondary pyoderma are frequent complications.

There may be no primary treatment for the diagnosed problem in which case palliative measures only are available and are required long term.

A definitive diagnosis may not be reached in which case palliative measures and control of secondary clinical signs are the only treatment option.

Chapter 7

Management of Diseases Presenting with Spots (Papules, Pustules, Vesicles and Bullae)

Papules are raised erythematous lesions 1–2 mm diameter caused by inflammation.

Pustules are raised erythematous lesions 1–2 mm diameter which contain inflammatory cells and are of two types.
- Sterile pustules are inflammatory cells alone
- Pustules contain inflammatory cells + bacteria which are indicative of infection

Vesicles (larger ones are bullae) are raised fluid-filled inflammatory lesions of variable size.

Epidermal collarettes are the end result of pustule formation.

Folliculitis is inflammation of the hair follicle. It may occur secondary to many inflammatory causes or may be the primary lesion in some immune-mediated diseases targeting on the hair follicle.

Papules, pustules vesicles and folliculitis can be indistinguishable on clinical examination.

A careful history and clinical examination, combined with laboratory investigations, especially cytology and histopathological examination are often required in all but the mildest and most transient cases.

Figure 7.1 outlines an approach to the investigation of diseases presenting with spots.

7.1 YOUNG ANIMALS

Young puppies frequently present with 'spots'. There are a number of different causes.

7.1.1 PUPPY STRANGLES

Puppy strangles can usually be recognised on clinical signs. There is an acute onset, often rapidly worsening pustular dermatosis of the muzzle, eyelids and pinnae, frequently with a very marked submandibular lymphadenopathy.

The puppy often presents with systemic signs and there can be rapid deterioration and death.

Pustules are usually sterile and although the prognosis is guarded, there is frequently a good response to glucocorticoids.

The cause is unknown.

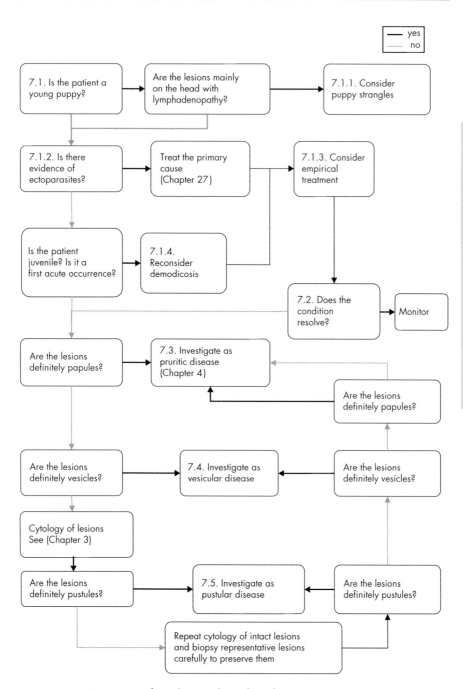

Figure 7.1 Management of papules, pustules and vesicles.

7.1.2   ECTOPARASITIC DISEASE

Ectoparasites should always be suspected in newly acquired puppies and young dogs, even in the apparent absence of pruritus or scale. The most common parasites are fleas and *Cheyletiella* spp., but lice also occasionally occur as a cause of papulo-pustular disease. Demodicosis is a very common cause of folliculitis in puppies and immature dogs (see Chapter 10).

7.1.3   MILD OR TRANSIENT CASES

Puppies frequently leave the litter with a mild ventral pustular dermatosis which responds to topical treatments only.

Juvenile pyoderma – before the skin immune system is fully mature young dogs are susceptible to ventral pustular dermatoses and also pustular lesions of the chin and muzzle. They are frequently recurrent but resolve by 2 years of age. Mild cases respond to topical treatments alone but more severe or persistent pyoderma may require systemic antibiotic therapy (Chapter 26.2).

Where lesions persist the possible underlying causes should be investigated.

7.1.4   DEMODICOSIS

Demodicosis should be ruled out before treating any young dog with pustular dermatoses empirically

7.2   SEVERE/RECURRENT OR PERSISTENT LESIONS

If the disease is of sudden and severe onset. it is important to obtain a definitive diagnosis quickly and in these cases cytology and biopsy may be indicated on the first visit.

For example, some cases of pemphigus or drug eruption present with severe lesions within a few days of onset and early definitive diagnosis is essential for successful treatment.

The first step is to ascertain whether the lesions are papules, pustules or vesicles. Any lesion containing liquid contents should be aspirated in a sterile manner and stained for direct microscopy.

Samples should be taken from intact pustules/vesicles at the same time for bacterial culture, identification and sensitivity testing.

See Chapter 3.

If in-house cytology does not identify the lesion, samples should be submitted to an external laboratory for further cytology and histopathological examination. Pustules and vesicles are usually very fragile, so care should be taken during the biopsy procedure to preserve the sample.

Excision biopsy may be preferable to punch biopsy, where shearing forces during rotation of the punch may tear the delicate lesion walls.

Management of Diseases Presenting with Spots

7.3 INVESTIGATION OF PAPULAR DISEASE

Persistent or recurrent papular disease should be investigated in the same way as pruritic skin disease (Chapter 4).

It is always important to distinguish papules from pustules, but this can be challenging on clinical signs alone.

7.4 INVESTIGATION OF VESICULAR DISEASE

Vesicles are an uncommon lesion in skin disease.

They frequently rupture before they are seen.

Intact vesicles should be aspirated for cytology.

Causes:

- Viral disease (Chapter 11.3)
- Immune-mediated disease (Chapter 13)
- Chemical and physical irritants

7.5 INVESTIGATION OF PUSTULAR DISEASE

Figure 7.2 outlines the investigation of pustular disease.

Acute responsive pyoderma (Chapter 26)
It has been said that healthy mature skin does not suffer from bacterial skin disease.

This is largely true, but if the underlying cause is transient and has resolved – reaction to shampoo, abrasion, pyotraumatic dermatitis, insect sting – a bacterial infection may persist for some time.

Mild to moderate pyoderma may require only topical treatment.

Moderate to severe pyoderma may also require systemic antibiotics.

Avoid glucocorticoids and other immune modulating drugs – acute moist dermatitis is an exception.

Glucocorticoid treatments may convert an acute responsive pyoderma into a chronic non-responsive pyoderma.

Persistent or recurrent cases
It is important at this stage to differentiate an infected pustule from a sterile pustule.

Figure 7.3 shows a sterile pustule. The neutrophils are minimally segmented and there are no intracellular bacteria. The cytoplasm has a uniform appearance.

Figure 7.4 shows an infected pustule. The neutrophils are multilobulated and there are bacteria in the cytoplasm. There may also be vacuoles in the cytoplasm.

Sterile pustules predominate
These conditions should be investigated as immune-mediated disease (Chapter 13).

Management of Diseases Presenting with Spots

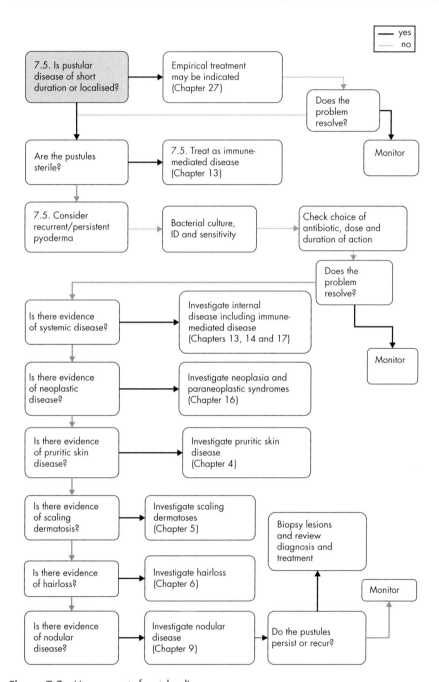

Figure 7.2 Management of pustular disease.

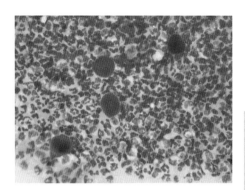

Figure 7.3 Sterile pustule with acanthocytes (courtesy of Nick Carmichael, CTDS Ltd).

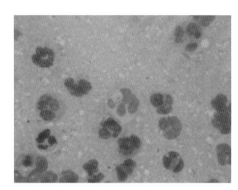

Figure 7.4 Neutrophils containing bacteria in a pustule (courtesy of Nick Carmichael, CTDS, Ltd).

Pyoderma

All cases of recurrent or persistent pyoderma should be investigated for an underlying cause (Chapter 11.1).

7.6 FOLLICULITIS

Folliculitis frequently accompanies papules, pustules and vesicles, and may occur in many inflammatory conditions.

Folliculitis is frequently only identified on histopathological examination.

The underlying cause should be identified and addressed.

Histopathology may also aid in identifying the underlying cause.

Cases of folliculitis should be managed carefully to avoid hair follicle rupture which may result in furunculosis.

The types of folliculitis and their underlying causes are listed in Table 7.1.

Luminal folliculitis
- Normally secondary to underlying causal factors
- Superficial disease affects mainly the infundibulum
- Severe deep disease affects all parts of the hair follicle causing destruction

Table 7.1 Types of folliculitis and their causes

Mild to moderate luminal folliculitis (secondary)	Micro-organism	Dermatophytosis Superficial bacterial folliculitis Miliary dermatitis
	Hypersensitivity	Flare factors
	Immune mediated	Pemphigus foliaceus Sterile eosinophilic pustulosis
Moderate to severe luminal folliculitis (secondary)	Micro-organism	Demodicosis Fungal kerion Canine and feline acne Acral lick dermatitis Interdigital furunculosis Callus pyoderma
	Immune mediated	Deep pyoderma/furunculosis Pelodera dermatitis Eosinophilic furunculosis of face (nasal pyoderma) Sebaceous adenitis
Mural folliculitis (primary)		Alopecia areata Demodicosis Pseudopelade Eosinophilic and granulomatous mural folliculitis in cats and dogs Follicular mucinosis

Mural folliculitis
- A large part of the follicle is targeted by a primary disease
- Can be characterised on histopathology
- Often immune mediated

Management of Diseases Presenting with Spots

Chapter 8

Approach to Changes in Pigmentation

There are many genetic and congenital causes of alterations to pigmentation, but they are rare and usually fairly readily recognised, such as albinism and breed associated conditions.

Acquired changes in pigmentation are more common and much more difficult to differentiate.

Where any change in pigmentation is accompanied by raised or ulcerated lesions, early biopsy is mandatory. Surgical excision with adequate margins should be performed in solitary lesions.

Figure 8.1 outlines the management of skin disease presenting with change in pigmentation. The numbers in the text refer to the numbers on the figure.

The changes in pigmentation can be an increase or a decrease or reddening of the skin.

8.1 CHANGES IN PIGMENTATION MAY BE GENERALISED OR MAY BE LOCALISED IN SPECIFIC PATTERNS

- Single discrete lesions
- Following patterns of disease, e.g. bilateral symmetry as in endocrine disease, or with a mucocutaneous pattern in some immune-mediated disease
- Multiple localised affected areas
- Hair follicle dysplasias where mainly the dorsum and trunk are affected

8.2 SECONDARY CHANGES IN PIGMENTATION SHOULD BE DIFFERENTIATED FROM PRIMARY CHANGES

- Erythema and also hyperpigmentation, which may occur secondary to inflammation or sunlight exposure in areas of hairloss

8.3 GENERALISED HYPERPIGMENTATION MAY OCCUR IN SOME ENDOCRINE AND NON-ENDOCRINE CONDITIONS

- Adrenal hyperplasia like syndrome (Chapter 14)
- Hyperadrenocorticism (Chapter 14)
- Hair follicle dysplasias (Chapter15)

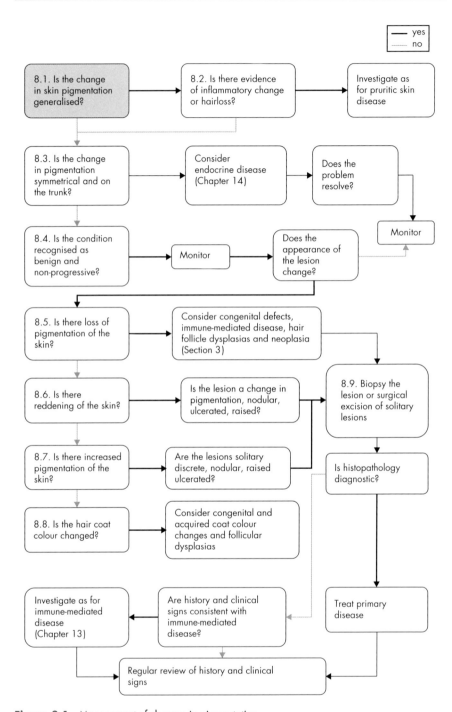

Figure 8.1 Management of changes in pigmentation.

Generalised loss of pigmentation is rare but may occur in some immune-mediated diseases. Congenital lack of pigmentation is seen in albinism.

8.4 PIGMENTARY CHANGE MAY BE BENIGN AND/OR TRANSIENT

Loss of pigmentation often occurs in:

- Scarring
- Idiopathic loss of nasal pigmentation in Labrador and golden retrievers and some other breeds

Hyperpigmentation is often seen:

- Lentigo simplex in the ginger cat where multiple macular lesions are seen on the lip and eyelid margins
- Hamartomas
- Macules, often secondary to inflammatory change
- Comedones can be mistaken for pigmentary change
- Inflammatory change, especially chronic inflammatory change

It is however important to biopsy representative areas when there is a change in pigmentation if it is not possible to confirm these benign changes as they are frequently associated with neoplasia.

8.5 LOSS OF PIGMENTATION OF THE SKIN

Less common than increase in pigmentation.

Differentiate from loss of pigment of the hair, which may accompany hypopigmented skin, or may occur on its own.

Biopsy should be performed at an early stage to rule out the possibility of neoplasia.

Causes:

- Scarring and idiopathic depigmentation
- Immune-mediated disease, e.g. vitiligo (Chapter 13)
- Neoplasia (Chapter 16)

8.6 REDDENING OF THE SKIN

This occurs most commonly in erythema.

To distinguish erythema from change in pigmentation (usually bleeding), press a microscope slide onto the skin. Blanching of the lesion indicates erythema, persistence of colouration indicates change in pigmentation.

Erythema most commonly occurs secondary to inflammatory disease.

Focal bleeding may occur in conditions which result in blood vessel fragility such as hyperadrenocorticism.

Telangiectasias are uncommon and usually benign. However, larger lesions may cause significant bleeding (Figure 24.2).

8.7 INCREASE IN PIGMENTATION

Normal pigmentary spots on pink skin and pigmented nipples must be differentiated from skin disease.

The most common cause of an increase in pigmentation occurs in inflammatory change (Chapter 4).

Hyperpigmentation is also common in endocrine disease (Chapter 14).

Biopsy should be performed at an early stage to differentiate benign lesions from neoplasia (Chapter 16) especially if the lesions are:

* Solitary or present as multiple discrete lesions
* Raised
* Ulcerated or inflamed
* Changing
* On the face or feet

8.8 LOSS OF PIGMENTATION OF HAIR COAT

A number of skin conditions may result in loss of pigment of the hair coat while the pigment of the skin remains unchanged.

* Temperature dependent acromelanism in the Siamese cat, which causes darker hair colouring at the extremities and may cause the hair coat to grow back darker after clipping
* Loss of pigmentation especially of the muzzle and periorbital areas in older dogs of some breeds
* Hair follicle dysplasias
* Idiopathic leukotrichia

These conditions are usually benign and are managed by supportive treatments alone where secondary complications cause irritation.

8.9 EARLY HISTOPATHOLOGICAL EXAMINATION IS ESSENTIAL

1   Where a solitary lesion can be removed it should be staged, examined cytologically where possible and excised with appropriate margins for definitive diagnosis and further treatment where necessary (Chapter 9).

Approach to Changes in Pigmentation

2 Where a solitary lesion cannot be removed, excisional or incisional biopsy for definitive diagnosis should be performed (Chapter 3).

8.10 SOME LESIONS CANNOT ALWAYS BE DEFINITIVELY DIAGNOSED ON BIOPSY

1 Immune-mediated disease frequently results in change in pigmentation. The history and clinical signs should be carefully reviewed (Chapter 13).
2 Some changes in pigmentation are not fully understood. The lesion should be regularly monitored for change.

Approach to Changes in Pigmentation

Chapter 9

Management of Raised and Ulcerative Skin Lesions

Figure 9.1 outlines the management of raised and ulcerative skin lesions. The numbers in the text refer to the numbers on the figure.

9.1 PAPULAR PUSTULAR AND VESICULAR DISEASE

Papular pustular and vesicular disease are described in Chapter 7.

9.2 EOSINOPHILIC GRANULOMA COMPLEX

The approach to these lesions of cats is described in Chapter 4.

The main raised lesions are:

- Linear granuloma
- Eosinophilic plaque
- Facial dermatitis
- 'Rodent ulcer'

It is important that these lesions are investigated at an early stage if the response to treatment is poor to differentiate from neoplasia and chronic infectious lesions.

9.3 CYTOLOGY OR HISTOPATHOLOGY

Depending on the lesion impression smears or aspirates for cytology or incisional biopsy for histopathological examination are useful in any raised or ulcerative lesion. The techniques are described in Chapter 3.

1 Impression smears are indicated in ulcerated or excoriated lesions
- The procedure is described in Chapter 3.4.
- Care should be taken in interpretation due to likelihood of surface contamination with micro-organisms.
- Where samples do not yield diagnostic information, biopsy or excision and histopathology should be performed.
- A provisional diagnosis of some neoplastic lesions, especially mast cell tumour, can be achieved in some cases.
- Neoplasia cannot be staged.
- Culture of open lesions does not yield useful diagnostic information, though cytology may.

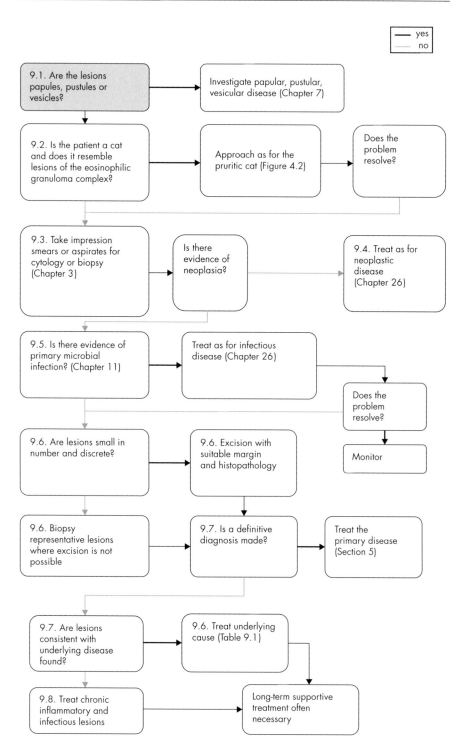

Figure 9.1 Management of raised and ulcerative skin lesions.

2   Fine needle aspirate is useful in any raised lesion
- The procedure is described in Chapter 3.
- The technique is susceptible to operator error.
- The yield of information can be increased in the hands of an experienced pathologist.
- Where results are inconclusive, biopsy or excision and histopathology should be performed.
- Where neoplastic lesions are identified staging, including biopsy or excision with histopathology should be performed.
- Fine needle aspirate before surgery can yield information regarding the margin of excision necessary by identifying the mass type but not the extent of the lesion.

3   Incisional biopsy is useful in any raised lesion
- Where excisional biopsy is possible this is preferable.
- An experienced dermatohistopathologist is essential.
- Staging is possible.
- Margins of excision cannot be determined.

9.4   TREATMENT OF NEOPLASTIC DISEASE

The treatment of neoplastic disease is described in Chapter 26.

9.5   RAISED LESIONS DUE TO MICRO-ORGANISMS

A number of skin diseases caused by micro-organisms can result in raised lesions. As well as raised inflammatory lesions such as bacterial granulomas, acral lick dermatitis, etc., occurring in many bacterial, yeast or fungal infections, there may also be raised primary lesions, for example:

- Fungal kerion
- Fungal or bacterial granuloma
- Poxvirus lesion
- Papilloma virus lesion

Other inflammatory lesions such as polyps of the ear canal and inflammatory gum lesions are also common.

These should be treated as described in Chapter 26.

Where a mass or small number of masses are well circumscribed and the anatomical area allows successful excision, histopathology should be achieved by excision biopsy with suitable margins. Where this is not possible incisional biopsy is indicated. Appropriate staging of the lesion should be done before this is attempted (Chapter 16).

9.6   DEFINITIVE DIAGNOSIS REACHED

Where neoplasia is diagnosed the lesion should be staged before a treatment plan is made.

Table 9.1 lists the main types of raised skin lesions and their underlying causes.

In some cases lesions consistent with a definitive underlying cause are found on biopsy, for example, calcinosis cutis in hyperadrenocorticism. In these cases the underlying cause should be investigated.

9.7 CHRONIC INFLAMMATORY AND BACTERIAL/FUNGAL LESIONS

These are extremely challenging to treat.

The underlying cause must be identified and addressed where possible.

The underlying cause may be obscured by the chronic inflammatory lesion.

Long-term supportive control is usually indicated.

Examples include:
- Eosinophilic granuloma complex
- Acral lick dermatitis
- Callus pyoderma
- Deep pyoderma/furunculosis
- Canine and feline acne

Table 9.1 Specific raised skin lesions

Lesion	Underlying causes	Characteristics
Calcinosis cutis and calcinosis circumscripta	HAC Dystrophic calcification	Often surrounded by inflammatory reaction. Hard tissue may resist biopsy
Hamartoma	Primary lesion	Proliferation of normal cells
Nevus	Primary lesion	Circumscribed developmental defect in skin
Granuloma	Bacterial, fungal, inflammatory	Nodular granulomatous inflammation
Furunculosis	Many inflammatory Often chronic	Often with deep pyoderma, resulting from foreign body reaction to imbedded keratin
Cysts	Usually idiopathic	Sac like structures with an epithelial lining
Hyperplasia	Many and diverse	Non-neoplastic proliferation of normal cells
Cutaneous horn	Many, may occur independently or associated with many tumour types	Warrants investigation of underlying cause
Neoplasia	Spontaneous Actinic Genetic factors Unknown factors	Variable, investigation mandatory

SECTION 3
AETIOLOGICAL APPROACH

Chapter 10

Diseases Caused by Ectoparasites

The common parasitic diseases of the companion animals are listed in Table 10.1.

10.1 DOG

10.1.1 FLEA BITE DERMATITIS (FIGURE 10.1) (ALSO SEE FIGURE 3.3)

Ctenocephalides felis
Ctenocephalides canis
Hedgehog flea rare
Rabbit flea rare

Table 10.1 List of common ectoparasites

Dog	Cat
Flea species	Flea species
Demodex canis	*Demodex cati, Demodex gatoei*
Sarcoptes scabiei	*Cheyletiella* spp.
Cheyletiella spp.	Ear mites *Otodectes cynotis*
Lice *Trichodectes canis*	Lice *Felicola subrostrata*
Lice *Linognathus setosus*	Ticks
Hookworm	Harvest mites
Ear mites *Otodectes cynotis*	(*Notoedres cati*) geographical variation
Ticks	(*Sarcoptes scabiei*)
Harvest mites	
Rabbit	**Ferret**
Fly strike – Myiasis	Flea species
Flea spp	Ear mites *Otodectes cynotis*
Fur mites – *Cheyletiella* spp.	Ticks
Listrophorus gibbus	
Ticks	
Ear mites – *Psoroptes cuniculi*	
Guinea pig	**Hamster**
Lice *Gliricola porcelli*	Demodex *D. criceti*
Trixacarus caviae	*D. aurati*
Gerbil	**Rat and mouse**
Ticks	Lice *Polyplax* spp.
Lice *Polyplax* sp.	Fur mites *Myobia* spp.
Mites	
Hedgehog	
Fly strike – myiasis	
Ticks	
Flea spp. *Archaeopsylla erinacei*	
Ear mites – *Otodectes cynotis*	

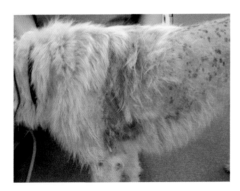

Figure 10.1 Dog with severe flea bite dermatitis.

Importance
- Most common cause of skin disease at some times of year
- Skin disease usually caused by hypersensitivity reaction to flea bite
- Relationship with other hypersensitivities
- Long-term ectoparasite control indicated
- Must be excluded before investigation for any other skin disease
- Cause of anaemia and debility in young puppies where there are heavy infestations
- Intermediate host of *Dipylidium caninum* tapeworm
- May be vector for other blood-borne diseases
- Zoonotic
- Cat fleas most common in the UK
- Dog fleas reported to be more common in rural Ireland
- Hedgehog fleas reports vary from common to rare in dogs
- Sessile rabbit fleas occasionally seen, causing pruritus of head and face
- Most common ectoparasite

Clinical signs
- May be asymptomatic
- Variable pruritus with or without lesions
- Most common presenting clinical signs dorsal hairloss with dorsal crusting lesions
- Also ventral papular and pustular rash seen, especially in young animals
- Chronic cases may result in widespread hairloss, hyperpigmentation and lichenification
- Face feet and ears usually spared

Diagnosis
- Single live flea sighting is significant
- Coat brushing for flea dirt, microscopy on suspicion (see Chapter 3)
- High index of suspicion on clinical signs
- A lack of evidence of fleas does not rule out flea bite dermatitis, especially in cats
- Allergy testing for flea antigen can be unreliable unless specific antigens, which may not be widely available, are used

Principles of treatment
Primary treatment (see Chapter 26.1)
- All in contact dogs and cats should be treated with insecticides with residual action
- Physical removal of life stages from environment by hoovering
- Environmental treatment in early stages at least
- Multi-animal households need year round aggressive flea control including environmental or life cycle treatment
- Fleas are a year round problem, still with seasonal peaks in many areas
- Thorough repeated aggressive flea treatment required to rule out involvement in skin disease

Supportive treatment (see Chapter 27.1)
- Glucocorticoids should be considered to break the itch–scratch cycle
- Up to 6 weeks treatment may be required to prevent recurrence of clinical signs

Topical treatments (see Chapter 29)
- As well as the primary treatments applied to the skin, shampooing is beneficial in removing fleas, scale and debris, reducing discomfort
- Shampooing should be timed so that ectoparasiticides are not removed from the skin

Outcome
- Good but long-term flea control usually required
- Guarded in severe cases where severe skin thickening, lichenification and deep pyoderma occur

10.1.2 CHEYLETIELLOSIS

Cheyletiella spp. (Figure 3.6)
Importance
- Common, especially in puppies
- Easily transmissible to other dogs, not demonstrated to other species
- May be asymptomatic
- Zoonotic

Diagnosis
- Clinical signs
- 'Walking dandruff' may be seen in heavy infestations
- Coat brushings with microscopy (see Chapter 3)
- Sellotape strips with microscopy (see Chapter 3)

Clinical signs
- May be asymptomatic
- Pruritus variably present
- Dorsal scaling frequently present

Diseases Caused by Ectoparasites

- Hairloss may be present
- Occasional ventral papular rash in young animals
- Papular rash on arms and abdomen of owner frequently found

Principles of treatment
Primary treatment (Chapter 26.1)
- Susceptible to most topical and systemic ectoparasiticides
- Treat in contact patients
- Treat beyond the length of the life cycle (3 weeks)
- Environmental ectoparasiticides
- Hot washing and tumble drying of bedding

Supportive treatments (Chapter 27.1)
- Glucocorticoids should be considered for 1–2 weeks to reduce patient discomfort

Topical treatments (Chapter 29)
- Shampoos are indicated to reduce patient discomfort and also to remove mites and eggs
- Local treatment of environment

Outcome
- Good as long in contact animals treated and source of infestation identified

10.1.3 SCABIES (FIGURE 10.2)

Sarcoptes scabiei var canis (Figure 3.7)
Importance
- Geographical variation in incidence, common to rare
- Urban fox population may be important
- May cause severe skin disease and intense pruritus
- Not susceptible to all insecticides
- Skin disease caused by irritant reaction to mite bites
- **Skin disease also caused by hypersensitivity reaction to mite and its faeces**
- Occasionally zoonotic

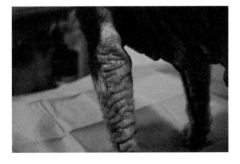

Figure 10.2 Cross breed dog with severe scabies.

Diseases Caused by Ectoparasites

Diagnosis
- History and clinical signs
- Skin scrapings are mandatory but lack of evidence of mites, eggs or faecal pellets does not rule out a diagnosis of scabies
- IgG serology available, more than 95% sensitivity and specificity reported
- Therapeutic trial with acaricide

Clinical signs
- Pruritus
- Erythematous papular skin disease
- Pinnae, elbows, hocks frequently first affected
- Often generalised ventral disease by time of presentation
- May cause lichenification, hyperpigmentation and skin folding in neglected cases

Principles of treatment
Primary treatment (Chapter 26.1)
- Multiple applications of effective acaricide
- Treat in contact dogs
- Environmental treatment may be used to prevent spread

Supportive treatment (Chapter 27.1)
- Intense pruritus warrants glucocorticoids throughout treatment period
- Pruritus may persist for 6 weeks beyond removal of live mites due to hypersensitivity reaction
- Consider pain relief in severe cases

Topical treatment (Chapter 29)
- Shampoos are indicated as it greatly improves patient comfort and removes mites and eggs

Outcome
- Good to guarded if clinical signs severe and skin disease chronic (Figure 10.2)

10.1.4 EAR MITES (FIGURE 3.9)

Importance
- Also affects cats and ferrets
- Common in young puppies
- Mite can survive outside the ear canal, aids transmission
- **IgE hypersensitivity reaction reported in cats**

Diagnosis
- Presence of mite demonstrated
  - May be seen on otoscopic examination
  - Microscopic examination of cerumen may demonstrate mites and eggs

- Evidence of mite
  - Age of patient and clinical signs
  - Dry crumbly altered cerumen
  - Otitis externa with other presentations
  - History of in contact affected dog, cat or ferret

Clinical signs
- Pruritus variably present
- Ceruminal discharge variably present

Principles of treatment
Primary treatment (Chapter 26.1)
- Susceptible to most acaricides
- Only use licensed topical preparations in the ears
- Ototoxicity of products used must be considered
- Treat all in contact dogs, cats and ferrets
- Poor targeting with topical acaricides due to presence of cerumen
- Poor penetration of systemic acaricides due to presence of cerumen
- Multiple treatments beyond the life cycle length (3 weeks) required

Supportive treatment (Chapter 27.1)
- Glucocorticoids should be considered where pruritus is severe
- Secondary bacterial or yeast otitis should be treated concurrently

Topical treatment (Chapter 29)
- Ear cleaning essential to remove mites, eggs and cerumen and to improve patient comfort

10.1.5   SKIN DISEASE DUE TO LOUSE INFESTATION (FIGURE 10.3)

Trichodectes canis (Figure 3.12)
Linognathus setosus (Figure 3.10)

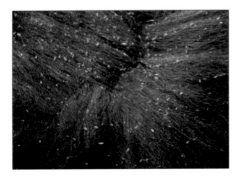

Figure 10.3 Scaling caused by louse infestation.

Importance
- *Trichodectes canis* most common, so skin irritation more common than anaemia
- Potential to cause anaemia in young puppies and severely affected animals in cases of louse infestation with the sucking louse *Linognathus setosus*
- Fairly common in young puppies and working dogs
- Not necessarily associated with poor environmental conditions
- Possible breed predisposition on hairy pinnae of spaniels
- Species specific

Diagnosis
- Lice are visible to the naked eye but may be hard to find
- Microscopy may reveal nits attached to hair, differentiate from *Cheyletiella* spp. eggs
- History and clinical signs

Clinical signs
- Pruritus usually present
- Variable dorsal scale
- Variable ventral papular rash
- Variable head-shaking and scratching
- Variable hairloss

Principles of treatment
Primary treatment (Chapter 26.1)
- Consider source of infestation, breeding and working kennels
- Treat all in contact animals of same species
- Adults susceptible to most ectoparasiticides
- Treat beyond the life cycle duration (3 weeks)

Supportive treatment (Chapter 27.1)
- Treatment with glucocorticoids for 1–2 weeks should be considered in pruritic cases

Topical treatment (Chapter 29)
- Shampooing is indicated for removing parasites scale and nits
- Patient comfort is increased and treatment duration may be decreased

Outcome
- Generally good, apart from in severe anaemia in young animals
- Reinfestation is common due to lifestyle (e.g. shooting dogs mixed while working)

10.1.6 HOOKWORM DERMATITIS

Importance
- Rare
- Generally restricted to earth runs in kennels
- Reaction to transcutaneous movement of endoparasite

Diagnosis
- History and clinical signs
- Demonstration of hookworm larvae

Clinical signs
- Restricted to feet

Principles of treatment
Primary treatment
- Review environment
- Endectocides treatment of all in contact of same species

Outcome
- Good to guarded if environmental factors not addressed

10.1.7   DEMODICOSIS (FIGURE 10.4)

Demodex canis (Figures 3.14 and 3.15)

Importance
- Relatively common in young animals of predisposed breeds
- Uncommon in adult dogs
- May be indicator or harbinger of immunosuppressive disease in adult onset
- Immunosuppressive disease not always present in adult onset, especially West Highland White Terrier and American Cocker Spaniel
- Can become life-threatening
  - Neglected or mistreated cases
  - Inadequately treated cases
  - Pododemodicosis
  - Generalised demodicosis
  - Generalised demodicosis with deep pyoderma

Diagnosis
- Deep skin scrapes of lesional areas
- Biopsy may be necessary to demonstrate mites in pododemodicosis or deep pyoderma

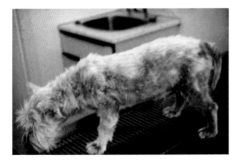

Figure 10.4   Westie with demodicosis.

Types of demodicosis
1 Juvenile onset localised
2 Juvenile onset progressive generalised
3 Pododemodicosis
4 Adult onset generalised progressive

Juvenile onset localised demodicosis
Clinical signs
- Discrete patches of hairloss
- Variable mild pruritus
- Localised pyoderma

Principles of treatment (see Table 10.2)
Primary treatment (Chapter 26.1)
- Systemic antibacterial therapy may be sufficient
- Do not use amitraz in toy breeds

Supportive treatment (Chapter 27.2)
- Do not use glucocorticoids in any circumstances. These should be withheld if being prescribed for other reasons. Careful liaison with other clinicians treating concomitant conditions is frequently necessary
- Concurrent systemic antibiotics and shampooing are indicated in all cases

Table 10.2 Principles of treatment of demodicosis

1 Avoid glucocorticoids and other immunomodulatory drugs in all cases
2 Consider pain relief in severe cases
3 Mild localised cases can be treated with supportive topical treatment (bathing) alone and monitored carefully for progression
4 Avoid amitraz in toy breeds
5 Careful coaching of clients where treatment to be done at home
  a. May cause sedation in operators
  b. Inadequate treatment or failure to follow instructions results in poor results
6 Generalised or progressive cases and cases of pododemodicosis should be treated aggressively
  a. Pre-wash with appropriate shampoo (Chapter 29)
  b. Use amitraz according to manufacturer's instructions
  c. Systemic antibacterial therapy throughout treatment
  d. Treatment beyond clinical cure
  e. Monitor response to treatment by live:dead ratio count of adult *Demodex* mites
7 Long-term treatment may be necessary
8 Recurrent cases may respond to repeated treatment
9 Other protocols for treatment in non-responsive cases can be considered, e.g. oral and topical avermectin and related treatments. This involves off label use of these products and is not without risk.
10 Use of ivermectin is contraindicated in Collies unless testing for the MDR1-gene defect is available

Topical treatments (Chapter 29)
- Shampooing indicated

Outcome
- Good unless progresses or inappropriately treated

Juvenile onset progressive generalised demodicosis
Clinical signs
- Generalised hairloss
- Discomfort or pruritus
- Generalised pyoderma
- Skin thickening, lichenification and hyperpigmentation

Principles of treatment
Primary treatment (Chapter 26.1)
- Amitraz according to data sheet indications indicated
- Systemic antibacterial therapy for duration of treatment
- Monitor response with live to dead ratio counts of mites

Supportive treatment (Chapter 27.2)
- Do not use glucocorticoids or other immunosuppressive drugs
- Consider pain relief

Topical treatment (Chapter 29)
- Degreasing shampoo should be precede each amitraz wash
- Clip long hair coats and consider clipping others
- Do not shampoo between treatments

Outcome
- Good but guarded if disease becomes progressive

Pododemodicosis
Clinical signs
- May exist as part of generalised demodicosis
- May occur in isolation
- Erythema, skin thickening, lichenification and/or hyperpigmentation of feet
- Variable pruritus/discomfort
- Variable hairloss
- Pyoderma

Principles of treatment
Primary treatment (Chapter 26.1)
- Amitraz according to data sheet recommendations indicated beyond clinical cure
- Systemic antibacterial therapy beyond clinical cure
- Negative skin scrapes do not indicate successful treatment as mites are hard to find on the feet. Continue treatment beyond clinical cure

- Treatment regimes using avermectins exist for non-responsive cases
- Systemic antibacterial therapy beyond clinical cure

Supportive treatment (Chapter 27.2)
- Glucocorticoids contraindicated
- Consider pain relief

Topical treatment
- Pre-treatment shampooing essential

Outcome
- Guarded, poor in recurrent and non-responsive cases

Adult onset progressive generalised demodicosis
Clinical signs
- Often history of glucocorticoid treatment
- West Highland White Terrier and American Cocker Spaniel predisposed
- May be concurrent systemic disease
- Erythema, skin thickening, lichenification and/or hyperpigmentation
- Variable hairloss
- Pyoderma

Principles of treatment
Primary treatment (Chapter 26.1)
- Identify underlying disease or predisposing drug where possible
- Amitraz according to data sheet recommendations indicated beyond clinical cure
- Systemic antibacterial treatment beyond clinical cure
- Monitor progress with live:dead counts of mites

Supportive treatments (Chapter 27.2)
- Glucocorticoids contraindicated
- Consider pain relief

Topical treatments (Chapter 29)
- Pre-treatment shampooing essential
- Selection of pre-treatment shampoo guided by clinical signs
- The choice of shampoo according to the type and severity of clinical signs is important

10.1.8 TICKS (FIGURES 10.5 AND 3.16)

Importance
- Vector for transmission of disease, e.g. Lyme disease, uncommon
- May result in local irritant reaction due to injection of tick saliva
- Granulomatous reactions which may require surgical excision may occur where mouth parts are left in situ

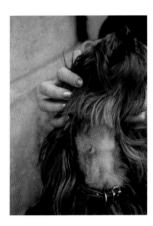

Figure 10.5 Tick bite granuloma.

Diagnosis
- Visible to the naked eye when engorged with blood

Clinical signs
- Variable irritation
- Localised granulomatous reaction

Principles of treatment
Primary treatment (Chapter 26.1)
- Physical removal of entire tick using proprietary tick remover
- Some topical ectoparasitides have repellent and/or early killing effects

Supportive treatment (Chapter 27)
- Not usually necessary

Topical treatment (Chapter 29)
- Topical steroid treatment may relieve temporary discomfort

Outcome
- Very good where no tick-borne systemic disease present
- Guarded where tick-borne systemic disease present
- Guarded where mouth parts are left in situ

10.1.9 HARVEST MITES (FIGURE 3.17)

Importance
- Prefer chalk soils, so rare to common depending on geographical location
- Skin disease induced by hypersensitivity reaction to third stage larvae

Diagnosis
- Mites are visible to the naked eye as bright orange dots
- Drop off or are removed by patient, so can be difficult to diagnose

Clinical signs
- Irritation of feet, especially toes with or without presence of mites
- Usually late summer

Principles of treatment
Primary treatment (Chapter 26.1)
- Insecticide sprays to kill mites if still present

Supportive treatment (Chapter 27.1)
- Glucocorticoids to reduce inflammation and pruritus

Topical treatment (Chapter 29)
- Not usually indicated

Outcome
- Good as long as self-trauma is limited

10.2   CATS

10.2.1   FLEA BITE DERMATITIS (FIGURES 10.6 AND 3.3)

Importance
- Most common cause of skin disease
- Skin disease usually caused by hypersensitivity reaction to flea
- Relationship with other hypersensitivity dermatitis
- Long-term flea control indicated
- Must be ruled out before investigation of any other skin disease
- May be challenging to find or rule out due to grooming habits of cats (see Chapter 4)
- Aggressive control methods often necessary to rule out presence of fleas
- May rarely cause anaemia and debility in young kittens in heavy infestations
- Intermediate host of *Dipylidium caninum*
- May be a vector of other blood-borne disease
- Zoonotic

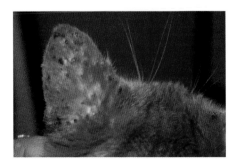

Figure 10.6   Rabbit flea bites on cat's ear.

Diagnosis
- Challenging
- Only clinical sign may be excess grooming which removes all evidence of fleas
- Grooming may be secretive even when excessive
- Recognition of pruritus
- Evidence of fleas
  1 Careful examination of the hair coat for fleas and flea dirt
  2 Gross examination of coat brushings with the owner present
  3 Microscopic examination of coat brushings
  4 Aggressive flea control with adulticides and insect growth regulators
  5 Microscopic examination of faeces for fleas
  6 Examination of coat brushings (gross and microscopic) from other animals in house
  7 Microscopic examination of hair for broken ends, indicating the presence of pruritus
  8 Full clinical examination of cat for evidence of overgrooming
    Hairloss, symmetrical or non-symmetrical
    Presence of lesions due to self-trauma
    Evidence of ectoparasites
    Presence of scale, crust, papules, etc.
    Microscopic examination of hair for broken ends
    Furball problems
    Fur attached to tongue papillae
    Presence of oral or lip 'granulomas'
    Faecal examination for hair, ectoparasites, etc.
  9 Review flea control
  10 Start to consider other diagnoses, but maintain flea control and monitor regularly

Clinical signs
- Cat fleas most common in the UK
- Dog fleas more commonly found in rural Ireland
- Hedgehog fleas variably reported
- Sessile rabbit fleas usually easily visible on face and ears, may cause pinnal pruritus and lesions, especially in hunting cats (Figure 10.6)
- May be asymptomatic
- May be pruritus with or without lesions
- Miliary dermatitis
- Feline symmetrical alopecia with little or no obvious evidence of underlying inflammation
- Eosinophilic granuloma complex
- Facial pruritus
- Pruritus may persist for several weeks beyond removal of parasite and is frequently self-perpetuating, especially in chronic cases

Principles of treatment
Primary treatment (Chapter 26.1)
- As diagnosis is challenging, aggressive treatment and ongoing control and prevention of fleas are essential in all feline skin disease
- Environmental treatment necessary at least in initial stages

- Residual flea treatments may need to be repeated more frequently in cases where overgrooming occurs
- Only products licensed for cats should be used for the treatment and control of and prophylaxis for fleas
- Constant review of flea control is essential in all feline skin disease
- Long-term parasite control of all in contact cats and dogs is essential for success

Supportive treatment (Chapter 27.1)
- Adequate control of pruritus is essential until and beyond the clinical resolution of lesions to prevent recrudescence
- Pyoderma secondary to FAD is uncommon, antibiotics are rarely indicated
- Consider glucocorticoids in pruritic cases
- Glucocorticoids indicated beyond clinical cure where skin lesions are present to prevent perpetuation by self-trauma
- Long-term glucocorticoid treatment may be indicated in severe cases and multi-cat households

Topical treatments (Chapter 29)
- May be of benefit but patient compliance usually poor

Outcome
- Can be challenging to control especially in multi-cat households

10.2.2 SCABIES

Importance
- Rare in the UK
- *Notoedres cati* infestation not reported in the UK since the 1960s
- *Sarcoptes scabiei* infestation may be associated with systemic disease

Diagnosis
- Clinical signs
- Demonstration of mite life stages or faeces on microscopic examination of superficial skin scrapings

Clinical signs
- Diffuse miliary dermatitis with scale and hairloss
- Variable pruritus

Principles of treatment
Primary treatment (Chapter 26.1)
- Investigate possibility of underlying systemic disease
- Monthly topical selamectin

Supportive treatment (Chapters 27.1 and 27.2)
- Treatment of underlying disease
- Consider glucocorticoids but care in the presence of underlying disease

Topical treatments (Chapter 29)
• Shampooing beneficial but patient compliance poor

Outcome
• Guarded due to likelihood of underlying systemic disease

10.2.3 CHEYLETIELLOSIS (FIGURE 3.6)

Importance
• Uncommon
• Presence of mites may be indicative of ageing or debilitated cats grooming less

Diagnosis
• Demonstration of mite on microscopy of coat brushings or sellotape strips

Clinical signs
• Variable pruritus
• Variable hairloss
• May be miliary dermatitis

Principles of treatment
Primary treatment (Chapter 26.1)
• Investigate possible causes of reduced grooming activity
• Acaricidal treatment according to data sheet recommendations

Supportive treatments (Chapter 27.2)
• Glucocorticoids may be indicated in severe cases
• Shampooing beneficial in removing parasites and eggs but patient compliance poor

Topical treatments (Chapter 29)
• Shampooing is always beneficial but not always possible
• Removal of parasite life stages decreases duration of treatment
• Improves patient comfort
• The choice of shampoo is dictated by the clinical signs
• Patients are frequently young, so milder shampoos should be chosen first

Outcome
• Good to guarded due to possibility of underlying disease resulting in reduced grooming

10.2.4 LICE

Felicola subrostrata (Figure 3.11)

Importance
• Uncommon
• May be indicative of ageing or debilitated cats grooming less

Diseases Caused by Ectoparasites

Diagnosis
- May be visible to naked eye
- Nits seen on microscopy of coat brushings

Clinical signs
- Variable
- Pruritus inconsistent
- Lesions inconsistent
  - Dorsal scaling
  - Mild hairloss
  - Miliary dermatitis

Principles of treatment
Primary treatment (Chapter 26.1)
- Susceptible to most ectoparasiticidal products
- Consider underlying causes of reduced grooming

Supportive treatment (Chapter 27)
- Shampooing would be beneficial in removing parasites, nits and scale

Outcome
- Good to guarded due to possibility of systemic underlying disease

Ticks are also seen in the cat and should be treated in the same way as in the dog.

10.2.5 DEMODICOSIS

Importance
- Rare
- May occur as harbinger of systemic disease
- May play a role in otitis externa, either as a primary or secondary factor

Diagnosis
- History and clinical signs
- Microscopy of deep skin scrapings
- Microscopic examination of cerumen

Clinical signs
- Variable
- Otitis externa
- Miliary dermatitis and scaling dermatoses

Principles of treatment
- Identify underlying disease or predisposing causes if possible

Primary treatment (Chapter 26.1)
- Amitraz is not licensed for use in the cat and is toxic
- Lime sulphur dips have been used off label with success

Supportive treatment (Chapters 27.2 and 27.3)
- Address underlying causes
- Symptomatic treatment of otitis externa

Topical treatment (Chapter 29)
- Lime sulphur dips off label may be primary treatment
- Caution with concurrent shampooing with other chemicals
- May be beneficial in improving patient comfort where possible

10.2.6   HARVEST MITES (FIGURE 10.7)

As for dogs, but even more frequently, the parasite may not be found on presentation. Significant pruritus and self-trauma due to hypersensitivity reaction is seen in predilected areas (face and feet).

10.3   RABBIT

10.3.1   FLEAS

Importance
- Vector for myxomatosis virus is main importance
- Myxomatosis usually fatal in unvaccinated rabbits
- Vaccinated rabbits may show clinical signs
- Rabbit does not need direct contact with wild rabbits for transmission of virus
- Flea bite dermatitis rare

Diagnosis
- Clinical signs of myxomatosis
- Sessile rabbit fleas may be seen on the head and ears
- Coat brushings may reveal flea dirt

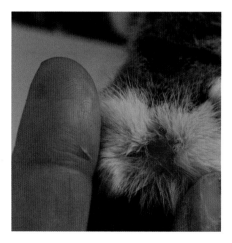

Figure 10.7 *Neotrombicula* causing discomfort between the toes of a cat.

Clinical signs
- Few attributable to flea bite dermatitis
- Myxomatosis

Principles of treatment
- Owner often unaware of risk of infestation
- Prophylaxis important in prevention of myxomatosis
  ○ Vaccination
  ○ Flea prophylaxis
- Environmental treatment necessary
- Prophylactic residual treatments necessary

10.3.2 *CHEYLETIELLA* (FIGURES 10.8 AND 3.6)

Importance
- Common especially in newly acquired rabbits
- Clinical signs may not be seen immediately
- Zoonosis

Diagnosis
- Clinical signs
- Microscopic examination of coat brushings/sellotape strips

Clinical signs
- Pruritus variable
- Lesions variable
- Dorsal scaling
- Localised severe scaling at the back of the neck
- Excessive moulting

Principles of treatment
Primary treatment (Table 26.10)
- Treat all in contact rabbits
- Environmental treatment or hutch cleaning

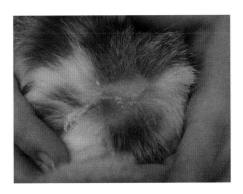

Figure 10.8 Scaling in a rabbit with cheyletiellosis.

- Topical or injected avermectins effective – off label use
- Treat beyond life cycle duration (3 weeks)

Supportive treatment (Chapter 27.1)
- Glucocorticoids may be used to treat pruritus – off label use

Topical treatments (Chapter 29)
- Generally shampooing not advisable due to stress caused to patient

Outcome
- Usually good though recurrence is common

10.3.3   FUR MITE (*LISTROPHORUS GIBBUS*) (FIGURE 3.18a)

Importance
- Fairly commonly found on coat brushings, clinical significance debatable
- Fairly commonly found in cases of mild pruritus, scaling and excess moulting were likely to be of clinical significance

Diagnosis
- Clinical signs
- Mite identified on microscopy of coat brushings or sellotape strips

Clinical signs
- Often none
- Variable pruritus
- Mild scaling
- Excessive or unusual moulting

Principles of treatment
- As cheyletiellosis (see Chapter 10.3.2)

Outcome
- Good if clinically significant unless systemic or dental disease is cause of undergrooming

10.3.4   EAR MITES (*PSOROPTES CUNICULI*) (SEE FIGURE 20.4)

Importance
- Uncommon
- Cause of severe pruritic otitis externa

Diagnosis
- Clinical signs
- Mite identified on microscopic examination of samples taken from crusting lesions

Clinical signs
- Pruritus
- Often associated with dorsal scaling dermatitis
- Severe erythematous otitis externa, inner pinna becomes lined with a honeycomb of crusting exudates

Principles of treatment
Primary treatment (Table 26.10)
- Removal of severe crusting lesions (see supportive treatment) essential
- Treat all in contact rabbits
- Use of topical or systemic avermectins beyond duration of life cycle (3 weeks) – off label use

Supportive treatment (Chapter 27.1)
- Softening and removal of excessive crusting exudates under sedation or general anaesthesia with perioperative pain relief
- Pain relief often required

Topical treatment (Chapter 29)
- Shampooing not usually advisable due to stress caused to patient
- Frequent ear cleaning to prevent further build up of exudates throughout treatment
- Symptomatic relief with off label use of glucocorticoid drops may be indicated

Outcome
- Guarded in severe chronic disease due to severity of otitis caused
- Good in mild cases

10.3.5 MYIASIS (FLY STRIKE)

Importance
- Very severe, often fatal
- Common disease of children's pets with inadequate care and environmental conditions
- Lack of awareness and inadequate parental supervision predispose
- Common with concurrent dental disease, dietary and digestive problems, where caecotrophs are not eaten or unpalatable to rabbit

Diagnosis
- Clinical signs
- Presence of maggots

Clinical signs
- Macerated flesh
- Presence of maggots
- Systemic illness
- Odour

Principles of treatment
- **Prevention is based on adequate husbandry, environment, diet and dental health**
- **Prophylactic treatment with topical cyromazine should be used where these factors are compromised**

Primary treatment (Table 26.10)
- Consider immediate euthanasia in severe cases
- Other than in mild cases, sedation and general anaesthesia are required to assess the severity of the disease and treat
- Physical removal of maggots and diseased tissues; consider euthanasia in severe cases
- Debride and clean

Supportive treatment (Chapter 27.2)
- Pain relief mandatory
- Fluid therapy and dietary support of very sick rabbit
- Frequent monitoring for hatching of fly eggs
- Secondary pyoderma and systemic infection usually required systemic antibacterial treatment in addition to topical therapy

Topical treatment (Chapter 29)
- Cyromazine as prophylaxis
- Chlorhexidine washes of affected areas
- Usually necessary but can cause fatality in stressed rabbits

Outcome
- Often difficult to evaluate the extent of the disease until examined under sedation/general anaesthesia, so guarded at outset
- Often fatal, so must be guarded to grave, except in mildest cases

10.4 GUINEA PIGS

10.4.1 SCABIES (*TRIXACARUS CAVIAE* INFESTATION) (FIGURE 3.19)

Importance
- Common
- Clinical signs may not occur until some long time after infestation
- Clinical signs may be related to stress
- Pruritic episodes and examination may induce fits, sometimes associated with collapse and death

Diagnosis
- Clinical signs
- Demonstration of mite on microscopy of superficial skin scrapes

Clinical signs
- Pruritus
- Erythematous excoriated lesions in areas easily scratched or nibbled

- Generalised hairloss, skin thickening, crusting
- Severe cases associated with weight loss and inappetence

Principles of treatment
Primary treatment (Table 26.10)
- Treat all in contact guinea pigs
- Topical or injectable avermectins – off label use
- Treat beyond life cycle of mite (3 weeks)

Supportive treatment (Chapter 27.1)
- Glucocorticoids may give short acting relief in severe pruritus
- Care when handling to avoid fits or collapse
- Shampooing may be beneficial but risk of stress is severe

Topical treatments
- Topical glucocorticoid preparations are usually removed by the patient and result in further self-trauma
- Shampooing should be avoided in pruritic guinea pigs to avoid stress and fits

Outcome
- Guarded in severe cases
- May be recurrent, especially in groups of guinea pigs

10.4.2 SKIN DISEASE DUE TO LOUSE INFESTATION (FIGURE 3.20a)

Importance
- Less common than scabies but may be difficult to differentiate on clinical signs
- Often asymptomatic

Diagnosis
- Lice demonstrated on microscopy of coat brushings, though visible to naked eye
- Clinical signs

Clinical signs
- Variable pruritus
- Mild to moderate dorsal scaling and hairloss
- May be asymptomatic

Principles of treatment
Primary treatment (Table 26.10)
- Topical or injectable avermectins – off label use
- Multiple treatments for 4–6 weeks usually required as biting lice are surface living

Supportive treatment
- Often not needed
- Consider glucocorticoids to control pruritus in severe cases

Topical treatments
- Not indicated and should be avoided in stressed and pruritic guinea pigs

Outcome
- Usually good

10.5 OTHER MITES AND LICE OF RABBITS MICE AND GERBILS (FIGURES 3.18b, 3.20b AND 3.21)

Importance
- Relatively uncommon as many animals are laboratory bred
- Variable clinical significance
- May be indicator of systemic disease causing reduced grooming
- Rabbit scabies has been reported more frequently in Mediterranean countries

Diagnosis
- Clinical signs
- Parasite demonstrated on microscopy of coat brushings or superficial scrapes

Clinical signs
- Variable pruritus
- Lesions not always present
- Mild cases may show mild scaling only
- Hairloss scale skin thickening and crusting

Principles of treatment
- Treat all in contact pets

Primary treatment (Table 26.10)
- Topical or injectable avermectins – off label use

Supportive treatment
- Not usually indicated or effective

Topical treatment
- Usually results in increased self-trauma

Outcome
- Usually good if patient and owner compliance good

Chapter 11

Skin Disease Caused by Micro-organisms

11.1   BACTERIAL INFECTIONS

Importance

A number of bacteria are of clinical significance in skin disease of which *Staphylococcus intermedius* or *pseudointermedius* is the most common and important. Most pathogenic organisms have been reported to be coagulase positive. It is rare for primary bacterial skin disease to occur in either the adult dog or cat, but secondary pyoderma is important and often challenging to treat.

The emergence of the meticillin resistant and sensitive staphylococcal species as a hospital acquired infection in human medicine has been mirrored by similar problems in veterinary medicine, although recent reports have suggested that the veterinary hospital acquired infections may cause slightly less severe disease, where removal of the initiating cause may often be curative. More recently, *Clostridium difficile* has produced similar challenges in treatment.

11.1.1   PYODERMA

'Healthy adult skin does not suffer from bacterial infection'.

This is largely true. There is usually a transient or persistent underlying cause. It is important to address the underlying cause in all recurrent or persistent cases of pyoderma.

Importance

Although rarely the cause of primary skin problems, consideration of pyoderma is very important in the treatment of skin disease.

- Secondary bacterial infection is common in most dermatological diseases.
- Once initiated secondary bacterial infection can be self-perpetuating even once the primary condition has resolved.
- Secondary bacterial infection can significantly contribute to patient discomfort.
- Control of secondary bacterial infection alone may be sufficient in some cases where the underlying cause is hard to address, e.g. hypersensitivity dermatitis
- Failure to treat bacterial infection may result in failure of treatment of the primary skin disease.
- The presence of a pruritic secondary pyoderma may mask a non-pruritic underlying cause, e.g. hypothyroidism.

Causes of bacterial skin infection

The normal immunological, chemical and physical barriers of the skin present an excellent defence against invasion by micro-organisms but any condition in which these defences are reduced may result in secondary pyoderma.

- Physical – trauma to the skin, including self-trauma, e.g. in pyotraumatic dermatitis
- Chemical – alteration of the constitution of the lipid layer, e.g. in hypersensitivity dermatitis, systemic disease
- Immunological – immune defect as in juvenile pyoderma, immunosuppression as in hyperadrenocorticism

The common causes of pyoderma are listed in Table 11.1.

Classification of pyoderma

- Surface pyoderma – e.g. acute moist dermatitis
- Superficial pyoderma – e.g. pyoderma secondary to hypersensitivity dermatitis
- Deep pyoderma – usually a progression from secondary pyoderma due to chronicity or severity, neglect or inappropriate treatment, often associated with furunculosis

Surface pyoderma

Importance
Most commonly caused by pyotraumatic dermatitis.

- Intertrigo – surface pyoderma in areas of friction (axilla, groin, tail base, neck folds) (Figure 11.1)
- Acute moist dermatitis (hot spot, wet eczema) – surface pyoderma often due to insect bite or other minor trauma resulting in rapid spread of lesion (Figure 11.2)

Diagnosis
History and clinical signs

Table 11.1　Common causes of pyoderma

Ectoparasites	e.g. demodicosis, scabies
Non-parasitic insect bites	e.g. fly bites
Fungal, viral and yeast dermatoses	e.g. dermatophytosis
Hypersensitivity dermatitis	e.g. flea bite dermatitis, atopic dermatitis
Endocrine disease	e.g. hypothyroidism, diabetes mellitus
Non-endocrine alopecias	e.g. colour dilution alopecia
Neoplasia, skin and systemic	e.g. lymphoma
Immunosuppressive disease	e.g. hyperadrenocorticism
Immunosuppressive treatments	e.g. glucocorticoids, cancer chemotherapy
Other immune-mediated disease	e.g. pemphigus foliaceus
Trauma and self-trauma	e.g. acute moist dermatitis, intertrigo
Immature skin immune system	e.g. juvenile impetigo, canine 'acne'
Metabolic disease	e.g. hepatic disease
Nutritional disease	e.g. zinc responsive dermatosis

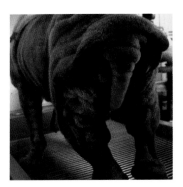

Figure 11.1 Intertrigo secondary to skin folding in a Sharpei.

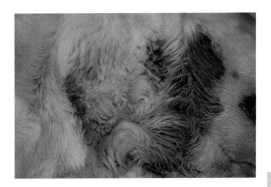

Figure 11.2 Acute moist dermatitis on a Labrador retriever.

Clinical signs
- Pruritus
- Acute onset lesion
- Erythema with marginal spread and hairloss
- Exudate usually present
- Labrador and golden retrievers and rottweilers predisposed, especially to facial lesions beneath the pinna

Principles of treatment
This is described in detail in Chapter 27.2.
1 All cases should be clipped free of hair and bathed using antibacterial washes beyond the margins of the lesion to prevent spread. Bathing twice daily should continue for several days to remove irritant exudates.
2 Anal sac disease and flea bite dermatitis are common underlying causes which should be investigated and addressed on first presentation.
3 Mild to moderate cases may respond to topical symptomatic treatment using anti-pruritic or antiseptic preparations and prevention of self-trauma alone.
4 Risk of progression to superficial and deep pyoderma especially in golden and Labrador retrievers and rottweilers if not treated aggressively and glucocorticoids are used.
5 Moderate to severe cases warrant additional systemic antibiotic treatment.
6 The underlying cause of persistent or recurrent cases should be investigated and addressed.
7 Glucocorticoids should be avoided in recurrent cases to avoid progression to superficial pyoderma.
8 Glucocorticoids should be avoided where progression to superficial or deep pyoderma is suspected.

Outcome
- Good as long as there is no progression to superficial or deep pyoderma
- More guarded in facial lesions of golden and Labrador retrievers and rottweilers
- More guarded where there is a persisting underlying cause

Superficial pyoderma (Figure 11.3)

Importance
- Very common as a significant secondary complication and flare factor in a number of dermatological diseases
- Underlying cause should always be investigated (Table 11.1)
- May mask underlying disease during investigation and treatment
- Inappropriate treatment may lead to deep pyoderma and furunculosis
- Superficial pyoderma should always be addressed and treated adequately

Diagnosis
- History and clinical signs
- Cytology of intact pustule
- Bacterial culture and identification
- Histopathology

Clinical signs
- Pustules (Figure 2.29)
- Papules (Figure 2.27)
- Epidermal collarettes (Figure 2.10)
- Inflammatory changes
- Hairloss
- Variable pruritus

Principles of treatment
Glucocorticoids are contraindicated.

Primary treatment
This is described in Chapter 27.2.
- Identify and address the underlying cause
- Topical treatment alone may be sufficient in localised or mild disease
- Systemic antibacterial treatment is indicated in chronic, recurrent, generalised or moderate to severe cases
- A suitable antibacterial agent can be chosen empirically in acute cases
- In chronic, recurrent or severe cases choice of antibacterial agent should follow bacterial culture, identification and sensitivity testing, although an empirical choice can be used until results are available to avoid delay in treatment

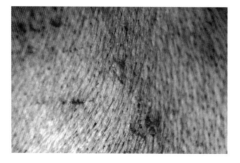

Figure 11.3 Pustules in superficial infection.

- The correct dose of the antibacterial agent should be used following accurate weighing of the patient
- The correct duration of treatment should be used
  - Acute mild cases 10–14 days, with review at the end of this time
  - First time more severe cases 3–6 weeks with review at the end of this time
  - Chronic, recurrent of severe cases, minimum 6 weeks and at least 3 weeks beyond clinical cure, with 3 weekly review to assess progress
- Long-term low dose and pulse dosing of antibiotic treatments have been used with some success in cases where the underlying cause is hard to address. They should not be used in short-term cases, and care should be taken to avoid regimens which may induce bacterial resistance.

Do not try to cut corners or costs in the choice of antibiotic, low dosing or short duration – it will cause frustration to owner and patient alike.

Supportive treatment
- Avoid systemic glucocorticoids
- Essential fatty acid and cofactor supplementation may increase patient comfort

Topical treatment
- Shampooing is always beneficial in removing irritant inflammatory products
- Antibacterial and antiseptic shampoos may reduce the duration of systemic treatment
- Antibacterial ointments may increase patient comfort where there are localised lesions and the patient can be prevented from licking

Deep pyoderma (Figures 2.15 and 11.4)
Importance
- Avoid progression to deep pyoderma by appropriate treatment of superficial pyoderma wherever possible
- Tends to be intractable to treatment and self-perpetuating even when underlying cause addressed
- Often associated with furunculosis, where keratin is dragged into the dermis by the inflammatory reaction and causes a persistent foreign body reaction. This provides a nidus of infection and also takes several months to resolve once all initiating factors have been treated. In practice this is often a permanent condition requiring lifelong management.

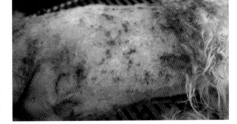

Figure 11.4 Deep pyoderma/furunculosis secondary to demodicosis in an adult American Cocker Spaniel.

Diagnosis
- History and clinical signs
- Bacterial culture and identification
- Biopsy

Clinical signs
- Pain or pruritus
- Systemic signs in severe cases
- Presence of draining tracts and fistulae
- Pustules
- Skin thickening, lichenification, erythema and exudation

Principles of treatment
This is described in Chapter 27.2.

- Identify and address the underlying cause
- Avoid glucocorticoids

Primary treatment (Chapter 26)
- Long-term appropriate systemic antibiotic therapy, at least 6 weeks beyond clinical cure
- May require several months or very long-term treatment with permanent control measures

Supportive treatment (Chapter 27)
- Identify and address systemic disease
- Pain relief
- Prevention of self-trauma and protection of excoriated and ulcerated areas

Topical treatment (Chapter 29)
- Shampoos always beneficial
- Care in choice of shampoo to avoid further tissue damage and discomfort
- Antibacterial ointments, gels and creams beneficial where removal by licking can be prevented
- Avoid antibiotic/glucocorticoid combinations

11.1.2 FURUNCULOSIS

Frequently persists after the resolution of deep pyoderma.

Remains challenging to treat even after addressing pyoderma and underlying causes.

Although glucocorticoids are contraindicated in the presence of deep pyoderma, systemic glucocorticoids may be the only way of controlling the persistent foreign body reaction and may be necessary to reduce patient discomfort.

If response to a trial period of glucocorticoids is good, long-term management is usually necessary.

11.1.3 LOCALISED PYODERMAS

These are described in Chapters 19–25.

11.1.4 HOSPITAL AND COMMUNITY ACQUIRED INFECTIONS

Meticillin resistant and sensitive staphylococcal infections (MRSA, MSSA, MRSI, MSSI) and *Clostridium difficile* are the most important infections reported.

Importance
- These can be either hospital acquired or community acquired infections
- Health and veterinary workers have a higher prevalence of carriage than the general population, so pets belonging to these groups of workers or recently hospitalised people should be considered at higher risk
- Hospital, isolation, hygiene and disinfection procedures are the most important factors in the prevention and management of these diseases
- These infections should be considered in any patient with pyoderma that does not respond to a single course of an appropriately used systemic antibiotic
- Post-operative wound infections and implant associated infections are at increased risk of being affected
- In urgent cases, the off label use of erythromycin has been effective while awaiting results
- Implant removal is often curative without the need for systemic antibiotics
- Guidelines for the prevention and control of these infections are available on the websites of the major veterinary organisations, e.g. BSAVA website www.bsava.com

Prevention and control
- High standards of cleaning and disinfection
- Hand washing and disinfection between patients and tasks
- Thorough cleansing of kennels and equipment between patients and at regular intervals during occupation
- Appropriate use of personal protective equipment to protect clinician and patient
- Segregation of waste according to regulations and infection risk and prompt disposal
- Appropriate and judicious use of antibiotics
- Infection control audits including environmental screening
- Consider staff screening with fully informed consent
- Sterilisation protocols employed for all instruments
- Disposable equipment where viable

Management
- Hospital acquired infections should be considered
- Slow or non-healing wounds
- Post-operative infections especially in the presence of implants
- Immunosuppressed patients
- Non-responsive skin infections

Isolation
- All waste should be treated as hazardous and segregated
- All equipment should be regarded as hazardous and processed separately

- Patients should be isolated and movement restricted within the hospital
- Barrier nursing using the minimum number of personnel should be instituted

Disinfection
- Hands
  - Washing for minimum 30 seconds using hot water and soap
  - Use of antibacterial hand washes, e.g. 4% chlorhexidine, 2% triclosan, povidone-iodine, 70% alcohol rub
- Environment
  - Lots of hot water and detergent to remove organic material
  - Disinfection with adequate contact time, e.g. 0.1% sodium hypochlorite, phenolic and aldehyde disinfectants are also effect but protocols for safe use should be in place
  - Drying and resting before re-use
- Patient
  - Wounds should be covered where possible
  - Antibacterial washes, e.g. benzoyl peroxide, 4% chlorhexidine with protocols for use for protection of staff handling patients

Treatment
- Treatment of primary problem
- Investigation of possibility of immunosuppression
- Removal of implants where possible
- Erythromycin can be used off label in urgent cases. Other antibacterials may be shown to be effective in particular environments
- Appropriate aggressive systemic antibacterial therapy following culture and sensitivity

11.1.5 RABBIT SYPHILIS

Caused by a spirochaete bacterium *Treponema cuniculi*. Relatively uncommon disease of mucocutaneous areas of rabbit.

Can be easily confused with mild cases of myxomatosis.

Difficult to achieve a definitive diagnosis, except on histopathology.

Responds to penicillins which should be used with caution in rabbits and all are used off label.

11.2 LEISHMANIOSIS

Importance
- Zoonotic, rare but serious and life-threatening disease can occur in man
- Common in Mediterranean Europe, this is an emerging disease in the UK. Euthanasia is compulsory or advised in some parts of the world due to risk to man

- Epidemiological surveys have shown prevalence of 1–50% exposure in some endemic countries
- Europe *Leishmania infantum* – vector *Phlebotomus* spp. Sandflies
- New world *Leishmania chagasi* – vector *Lutzomyia* spp. Sandflies
- Local knowledge useful for avoidance of the vector

Diagnosis

Diagnosis is made on the basis of clinical signs and history of exposure, positive serology (using IFA and PCR) and isolation of parasites from lymph node smear, as well as positive skin test results.

Treatment

The standard internal medicine texts should be consulted for the treatment of leishmaniosis. Allopurinol should not be used alone as it may result in the persistence of parasite life stages. Allopurinol, aminosidine, azoles, pentamidine or lomidine and amphotericin B.

Prevention

- Prevent biting by sandflies, by avoiding late afternoon walks to infested areas
- Insecticides to reduce number of sandflies in affected areas
- Fly repellants and insecticides on the pet

Uncommon and rare bacterial skin diseases

Some of these diseases are more important because of their systemic effects than for the skin diseases they cause. Relevant internal medicine texts should be consulted for the most up to date information.

- Bacterial granulomas
- Feline leprosy
- Actinomycosis
- Actinobacillosis
- Nocardiosis
- Streptococcal and staphylococcal necrolising fasciitis – toxic shock syndrome
- Brucellosis
- Plague
- Lyme borreliosis
- Listeriosis
- Rabbit syphilis

11.3 FUNGAL INFECTIONS

Fungal infections are most important in warm and humid climates.

All nodular and ulcerative lesions and draining tracks should be investigated for the presence of fungal infections.

Contamination of wounds with geophilic fungal species can result in skin lesions as well as parasitic species.

11.3.1   DERMATOPHYTOSIS

'If it looks like ringworm it probably isn't'.

- Fungal infection of keratin structures of the skin – hair and nails
- Migrates as far as the zone of keratinisation (Adamson's fringe)
- Aided by fungal production of keratolytic enzymes
- Infected hairs grow out and break off, resulting in hairloss
- Caused by dermatophilic organisms

Cats
Microsporum canis – most common

Also *Trichophyton mentagrophytes, Trichophyton verrucosum, Microsporum gypseum* and *Microsporum persicolor*

Importance
- Prevalence in domestic cats with consistent dermatological lesions 30% – panEuropean study
- Higher frequencies in autumn and winter
- Carrier state and infection major problem in catteries and showing and breeding colonies
- Zoonosis
- Once diagnosed, in contact cats cannot be shown until three clear consecutive cultures are obtained

Diagnosis
- History and clinical signs (strong predisposing factors)
  - Kittens and cats less than 1 year old
  - Pregnant and lactating queens
  - Cats in breeding colonies and cats
  - Longhaired pedigree cats
  - Old and immunosuppressed cats
  - Pre-existing inflammatory disease may predispose
- Direct microscopy – false negatives are common unless very experienced technicians
- Woods Lamp examination (Figure 11.5)
  - Useful screening test but only 50% of *Microsporum canis* fluoresces and most other species do not
  - Ultraviolet light of specific wavelength essential
- **Dermatophytosis cannot be ruled out on Woods Lamp examination**
- Fungal culture
  - Definitive diagnosis on appropriate medium
  - Colour change
  - Colony appearance
  - May take up to 6 weeks
- Histopathology
  - Experienced dermatopathologists may detect on routinely stained preparations
  - PAS stains demonstrate fungal hyphae
- Owner lesions (Figure 3.24)

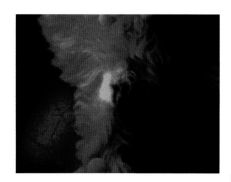

Figure 11.5 Dermatophytosis lesion fluorescing under Woods Lamp.

Clinical signs
- Asymptomatic carrier state common
- Pruritus variable to mild
- Hairloss
- Scaling
- Occasionally discrete lesions, especially kittens

Principles of treatment
This is described in Chapter 26.2.1.

Primary treatment (Chapter 26)
- Separate cats from any immunocompromised humans
- Glucocorticoids and other immunosuppressive drugs are contraindicated
- Investigate possibility of immunosuppressive disease
- Treat all in contact cats and close colony
- Environmental treatment essential
- Itraconazole licensed for use in cats and effective

Supportive treatment (Chapters 27.2 and 27.3)
- Clip and bathe persistent/recurrent kittens

Topical treatment (Chapter 29)
- Chlorhexidine/miconazole shampoos licensed for use and beneficial in reducing spread and increasing patient comfort where compliant
- Creams, gels and ointments rarely effective and usually groomed off
- **Enilconazole is toxic to cats**
- Griseofulvin is probably not indicated in the presence of a licensed alternative

Outcome
- Good in single cat households and kittens
- Guarded in showing and breeding colonies

Dogs
Importance
- Much less common than in cats
- *Microsporum canis* most common

- Also *Trichophyton mentagrophytes, Microsporum gypseum,* occasionally other *Trichophyton* species
- Higher frequencies in autumn and winter
- Can be zoonotic, but dog is end host for most species, so transfer is less common than cat

Diagnosis
- As for cats

Clinical signs (Figure 11.6)
- May be very varied or asymptomatic
- Lesions mainly head, ears, tail and paws, but may affect body
- Multiple patches of hairloss and scaling with minimal erythema most commonly
- Other presentations
  ○ Pruritus
  ○ Miliary dermatitis
  ○ Papules and pustules
  ○ Paronychia
  ○ Chin furunculosis
  ○ Nodules

Principles of treatment
Primary treatment (Chapter 26.2.1)
- Glucocorticoids and other immunosuppressive drugs are contraindicated
- Separate all animals from immunocompromised humans
- Treat all in contacts though spread less likely in the dog
- Treat or remove the source
- Itraconazole – off label use; effective and supporting data
- Griseofulvin – off label use. This is probably not indicated due to greater efficacy and operator safety of itraconazole

Supporting treatment (Chapters 27.2 and 27.3)
- Clip and bathe coat in recurrent/persistent cases
- Clip and bathe lesions

Topical treatment (Chapter 29)
- Chlorhexidine/miconazole shampoos
- Creams and ointments usually ineffective except in very localised lesions where removal can be prevented

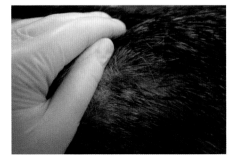

Figure 11.6 Dermatophytosis lesion on a Border Terrier.

Outcome
- Generally good, guarded if source of infection not established and addressed

Small animals
Importance
- *Trichophyton mentagrophytes* most important species
- Hairloss, scaling, mild pruritus
- Important as often unsupervised handling by children
- **Commonly zoonotic, especially children and immunosuppressed individuals**

Diagnosis
- Often challenging as children's pets and diagnostic investigations can be expensive
- Fungal culture

Clinical signs
- Localised lesions
- Generalised mild scaling
- Generalised hairloss
- Mild inflammatory change
- Pruritus mild to absent without secondary pyoderma
- Chronic cases where inflammation and pruritus are significant are often presented on Saturday mornings

Principles of treatment
Primary treatment (Chapter 26.2.1)
- Consider euthanasia in children's pets because of zoonotic risk
- Itraconazole – off label use; effective and data to support use
- Treat all in contacts
- Environmental treatment
- Off label use of griseofulvin inadvisable due to risk of handling, especially small doses

Supportive treatment (Chapter 27)
- Clip and bathe in chronic cases

Topical treatments
- Avoid as shampooing increases operator risk and stresses patient

Outcome
- Guarded

11.3.2 OTHER FUNGAL INFECTIONS

- Uncommon
- Fungal mycetoma
- Fungal kerion
- Phaeohyphomycosis
- Sporotrichosis

- Blastomycosis
- Cryptococcosis

11.4 *MALASSEZIA* DERMATITIS

'*Malassezia* dermatitis is usually a secondary flare factor of inflammatory or non-inflammatory skin disease'.

Important cause of skin disease in dogs, cats and rabbits.

11.4.1 DOGS

Importance
- Common
- Normal cutaneous flora of the dog *Malassezia pachydermatis*, also M. *furfur* and M. *obtusa* in the external ear canal, also occasional reports of M. *sympodialis*
- Host responses: non-specific phagocytosis, specific cell-mediated responses, multiplication of epidermal cells, resulting in increased scaling and hence increased rate of removal of the organism

Malassezia dermatitis results from:
1   Increased numbers of *Malassezia* due to:
    increased humidity of skin
    increased or abnormal sebum production (cerumen in ear canals)
    damage to epidermal barrier
    folding of skin
2   Hypersensitivity response to *Malassezia* organisms

Diagnosis
- Clinical signs
- Microscopy of impression smears, tape strips, etc.
- Microscopy of cerumen (>10 yeasts per HPF indicative of disease)
- Culture
- Histopathology

Clinical signs
- Predisposed breeds, West Highland White Terrier, Basset Hound, English Settter, Shih Tzu, Dachshund, English Cocker Spaniel, American Cocker Spaniel and some others
- Early signs include erythema, pruritus and scaling
- Progresses to lichenification and hyperpigmentation with strong rancid fat odour
- Affects ventral neck, axillae, inguinal and perianal regions
- Spreads to affect neck, head, legs
- Often concurrent ceruminous otitis externa

Principles of treatment
Primary treatment (Chapter 26.2.1)
- Identify and address underlying cause
- Long-term control is usually required unless underlying cause can be cured

- Topical treatments usually used initially
- Systemic treatment with itraconazole or ketoconazole is occasionally required

11.4.2 CATS

Importance
- Uncommon in the cat
- Possible that breeds with abnormal fur are predisposed
- *Malassezia pachydermatis, M. globosa, M. sympodialis* and *M. furfur*
- In the cat, *Malassezia* dermatitis has been seen in FIV positive animals and secondary to thymoma and pancreatic adenocarcinoma

Diagnosis
- As for dogs (Chapter 11.3.1)

Clinical signs
- Generalised scaling and greasiness
- Ceruminous otitis externa
- Facial dermatitis in short nosed breeds

Principles of treatment
Primary treatment (Chapter 26.2.1)
- Identify and address underlying cause
- Long-term control is usually required unless underlying cause can be cured
- Topical treatments usually used initially, but more challenging in the cat
- Systemic treatment with itraconazole or ketoconazole is occasionally required
- **Enilconazole is toxic to cats**

11.4.3 RABBITS

Importance
- Uncommon
- Less is known about the disease in rabbits

Diagnosis
- As for dogs and cats (Chapter 11.3.1)

Clinical signs
- Pruritus mild to absent
- Generalised scaling
- Mild hairloss

Principles of treatment
Primary treatment (Chapter 26.2.1)
- Topical treatments less well tolerated in rabbits
- Itraconazole – little information available

Supportive treatment (Chapter 27)
- Address possible underlying causes especially ectoparasitic disease and dental and dietary problems where grooming may be reduced

Topical treatments (Chapter 29)
- Care in use, toxicity may be higher due to grooming habits of rabbits
- Chlorhexidine/miconazole shampoos but may be stressful

11.5   SKIN DISEASES CAUSED BY VIRUSES

11.5.1   DISTEMPER

Systemic disease may be accompanied by crusting hyperplastic lesions of the footpads and nasal planum.

11.5.2   POX VIRUS

Should be included in the list of differential diagnoses in feline nodular disease.

May be associated with immunosuppressive disease or treatment.

Diagnosis usually made on clinical signs and histopathology.

11.5.3   PAPILLOMA VIRUS

Causes multiple verrucose lesions, usually around the mouth or eyes.

May resolve spontaneously or be surgically removed.

11.5.4   FIV ASSOCIATED SKIN LESIONS

This is rare and controversial.

11.5.5   MYXOMATOSIS

Importance
- An important disease of both wild and domesticated rabbits
- Many owners underestimate the exposure of their rabbit to the virus
- Rabbit flea is the main vector

Clinical signs
- Severe systemic illness accompanied by severe mucocutaneous swelling, ulceration and discharge. Most commonly fatal (see Figure 21.4)
- Some vaccinated animals may demonstrate a more benign form of the disease which is more amenable to treatment, usually supportive

Diagnosis
- Clinical signs and history

Prevention
- Six monthly vaccination in high risk areas, annual vaccination in low risk areas
- Flea control and separation from wild rabbits in affected areas

Treatment
- Supportive treatment only is available
- Vaccination of in contact rabbits

Chapter 12

Hypersensitivity Dermatitis

Hypersensitivity dermatitis is the most common cause of skin disease in the dog and cat. It is still relatively poorly understood in these species and even less is known about the disease in the smaller mammals.

Hypersensitivity dermatitis may occur as a reaction to a single allergen or group of allergens such as pollen allergies in atopic dermatitis. However, a more complex situation occurs in many cases. There is evidence that, although the susceptibility to hypersensitivity is inherited via the MHC complex, the allergens to which patients react is based on their environmental experience. It is also recognised that, dogs with atopic dermatitis are more susceptible to flea bite dermatitis. Other associated links may be identified in the future. One allergen or group of allergens may be insufficient to trigger a pruritic dermatitis and so the concept of the pruritic threshold may explain intermittent, recurrent dermatitis often seen in hypersensitivity. Figure 12.1 shows how this may occur.

Hypersensitivity dermatitis is largely a diagnosis of elimination. Figure 12.2 describes the steps in this process, many of which are the same as those described in Chapter 4.

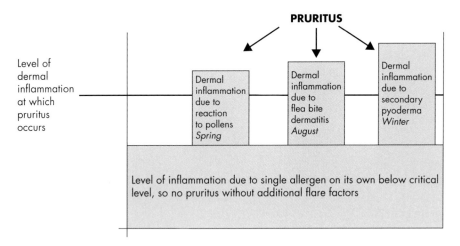

Figure 12.1   Pruritic threshold.

12.1   PARASITIC HYPERSENSITIVITY

Importance
- Often the most common type of hypersensitivity due to the prevalence of hypersensitivity reaction to flea saliva antigens

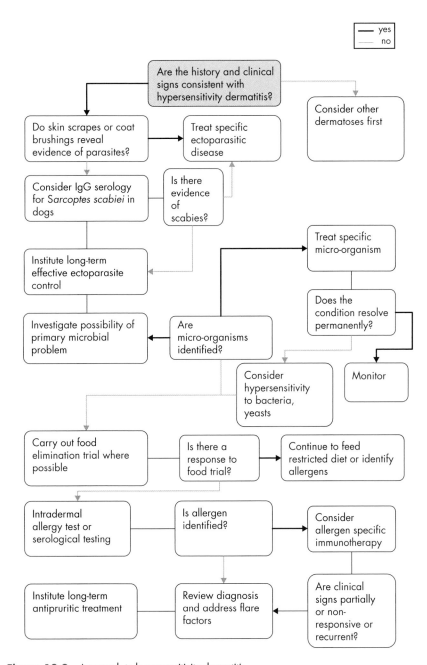

Figure 12.2 Approach to hypersensitivity dermatitis.

- *Sarcoptes* hypersensitivity and *Otodectes* hypersensitivity also important
- A small number of parasites result in a disproportionate amount of irritation
- Often mimics atopic dermatitis and cutaneous adverse reaction to fleas
- Important to rule out before investigating other causes of hypersensitivity dermatitis

Diagnosis
- Demonstrate presence of parasite life stages or faeces on microscopy of coat brushings, cerumen samples or skin scrapes
- IgG serological test for scabies
- Flea antigen tests variably sensitive and specific depending on antigens used
- Response to treatment with appropriate insecticides and acaricides
- Clinical signs
- Supportive histopathology often with predominance of eosinophils in dermal cellular infiltrate

Clinical signs
- See Chapter 10 for clinical signs specific to hypersensitivity to each parasite

Principles of treatment
Primary treatment
- Remove ectoparasites using appropriate acaricide or insecticide (Chapter 26.1)
- For flea bite dermatitis long-term control is necessary to avoid overuse of antipruritic treatments
- In multi-animal household long-term antipruritic therapy may be necessary for animals sensitive to flea saliva antigens as parasite control alone may be inadequate

Supportive treatment
- Treat secondary pyoderma (Figure 12.3) (Chapter 27.2)
- Antipruritic therapy always necessary in early stages (Chapter 27.1)
- Antipruritic therapy may be necessary long term
- Dietary supplementation (Chapter 27.2)

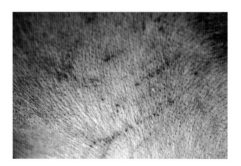

Figure 12.3 Secondary pyoderma in hypersensitivity dermatitis.

Topical treatments
- Always beneficial in increasing patient comfort and decreasing parasite load
- Avoid washing off topical preparations with residual action
- Choice of shampoo depends on clinical signs (see Chapter 29)

12.2 ATOPIC DERMATITIS

Importance
- The most common cause of hypersensitivity dermatitis at some times of the year

- Very common, possibly increasing – though may be due to increased recognition by veterinary surgeons, awareness by owners and hence increased diagnostic investigations
- Inherited predisposition MHCII
- Damage to the physical, chemical and immunological barriers of the epidermis is now thought to be a primary event
- Once thought to be due to inhalation of environmental allergens but now significant evidence for transcutaneous passage of allergens facilitated by the damage to the epidermal barrier
- Results in activation of antigen presenting cells (Langerhans cells) and Mast cells which leads to inflammatory cell infiltration in the dermis with Th2 cytokine expression

Chronic atopic dermatitis
- There is thought to be a switch from Th2 to Th1 cytokine expression, which allows self-perpetuation of dermatitis. Self-trauma results in increased access to allergens and micro-organisms
- Staphylococci produce superantigens which further active mast cells
- Keratinocytes and mononuclear cells activated, resulting in further inflammatory mediator release
- Lack of resolution of primary inflammatory event due to cascade of release of inflammatory mediators
- Self-antigens may be produced so that further stimulation by external environmental allergens is not necessary to perpetuate the inflammation

Diagnosis
- History
  - Peak age range between 1 and 3 years, but many cases presented outside this range
  - Age cannot be used to exclude diagnosis
  - Breed predispositions (Table 12.1)
- Clinical signs
- Elimination of other causes of pruritus (Chapter 4)

Table 12.1 Breed predisposition to atopic dermatitis (according to various reports in the literature worldwide)

American Cocker Spaniel	Miniature Schnauzer
Boxer*	Poodle
Bull Terriers*	Pug
Cairn Terrier*	Pyrenean Shepherd Dogs
Chihuahua	Scottish Terrier*
Dalmatian	Setter
English Bulldog	Tervuran Shepherd Dogs
German Shepherd Dog*	West Highland White Terrier*
Golden Retriever*	Wire Haired Fox Terrier*
Labrador Retriever*	Yorkshire Terrier
Lhasa Apso	

*Cited twice or more

Hypersensitivity Dermatitis

- Supportive histopathology
- Supportive intradermal allergy test (Figure 12.4) or serological test

Clinical signs
- Pruritus, erythema and hairloss
- Pruritus is usually moderate unless complicated by flare factors in which case can be severe
- Generally less pruritic than parasitic dermatitis
- Commonly involves feet, face and ears
- Periorbital erythema and hairloss
- Inflammation of axillae and groin
- Pinnal erythema – may be only clinical signs
- Pododermatitis
- Cheilitis
- Secondary ventral papular or pustular rash

Principles of treatment
Primary treatment (Chapter 26.3)
- ASIT treatment of choice
- All other treatments aimed at reducing pruritus
- Prednisolone or methylprednisolone
- Cyclosporine
- Herbal supplements
- Essential fatty acids
- Antihistamines
- (Tricyclic antidepressants and leukotrienes have also been used)

Supportive treatment (Chapter 27.1)
- Treat flare factors
- Yeast infections – chlorhexidine/miconazole shampoos
- Bacterial infections – systemic and topical antibacterial treatments
- Parasite control – predisposed to flea bite dermatitis
- Dietary supplementation may be beneficial

Topical treatments
- Shampooing always beneficial
- Choice of shampoo based on clinical signs to control erythema, pruritus, scale, flare factors, secondary inflammation (Chapter 29)

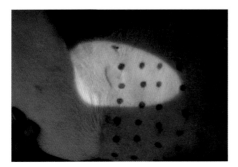

Figure 12.4 Positive reaction to intradermal test.

- Gels, ointments and creams not usually indicated except in very localised lesions where self-trauma can be controlled
- Glucocorticoid sprays may be indicated for localised lesions
- Glucocorticoid eye drops for related conjunctivitis

12.3 ADVERSE CUTANEOUS REACTION TO FOOD

Importance
- Aetiopathogenesis not fully understood
- Reactions to food can be caused by:
  - Response to foods containing high amounts of histamine
  - Hypersensitivity reaction
  - Non-allergic based intolerance to foods
- Prevalence unknown due to difficulties in diagnosis
- Some authors report common
- Diagnosis may be masked by concurrent atopic dermatitis
- Should be distinguished from increased dietary requirements occurring in pruritic skin diseases
- Can be clinically indistinguishable from other hypersensitivity dermatitis
- No evidence to support "accepted wisdoms" used to distinguish from other hypersensitivity dermatitis
  - Not necessarily more common in patients 6–12 months than atopic dermatitis
  - Not necessarily related to facial or perianal lesions
  - Not necessarily associated with a predominance of eosinophils in dermal cellular infiltrate
  - Not necessarily less responsive to glucocorticoid therapy
- May be associated with gastrointestinal signs

Diagnosis – testing for adverse reaction to food
Figure 12.5 outlines the investigation of suspected adverse cutaneous reaction to food.

- The gold standard test for adverse reaction to food remains the 12 week home-cooked diet using a novel protein source and a novel carbohydrate source with no additives, but it is increasingly difficult for busy clients to cook for their dogs and cats
- Hydrolysed diets of restricted molecular weights are frequently used as a useful compromise solution where it is not possible to use a home-cooked diet
- Commercial restricted protein source diets may contain trace quantities of other proteins which may trigger an adverse food reaction resulting in failure of food trials
- The use of intradermal allergen testing and in vitro serological testing for specific IgG and IgE cannot be used alone in diagnosis or exclusion

The incidence of cutaneous adverse reaction to food is unknown due to:
- No availability of simple single reliable diagnostic test
- Poor owner and pet compliance in food elimination trials
- Wrong choice of protein and carbohydrate sources
- Processing or additions to commercial diets may cause trial failure

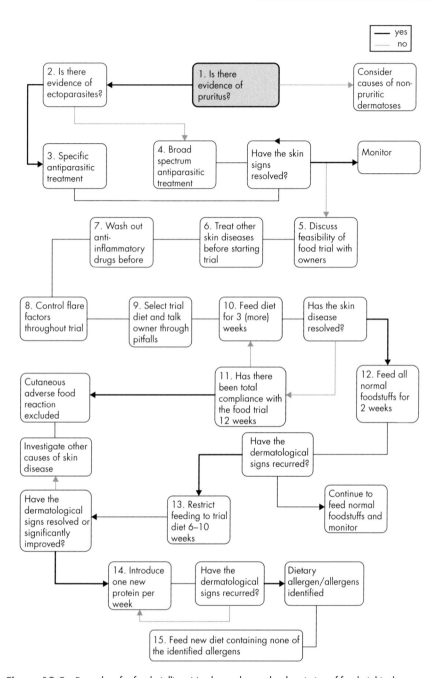

Figure 12.5 Procedure for food trialling. Numbers relate to the description of food trial in the text.

- Insufficient time given for food elimination trial
- False negative and false positive results of food allergy serological tests
- Concomitant pruritic skin diseases, with pruritus due to food adverse reaction partly contributing (see Figure 12.1)

Hypersensitivity Dermatitis

If a food elimination trial cannot be done properly, don't do it at all.

Tests available:

1 Home-cooked food elimination trial using a novel protein source and novel carbo-hydrate source
2 Food elimination trial using a commercial restricted protein diet
3 Food elimination trial using a hydrolysed diet (all proteins and carbohydrates below MW 9000)
4 Intradermal test to food allergens
5 IgG and IgE serological tests

The many 'hypoallergenic' diets available in pet shops and supermarkets are not suit-able for food elimination trials as they are not tailor made for the selection of novel proteins in the individual patient. Hydrolysed diets are an acceptable alternative.

The instructions for conducting a food elimination trial below are comprehensive and should be followed in their entirety. Some compromises may be necessary but the own-ers should be made aware of this. It should be read in conjunction with the flow chart (Figure 12.5). The numbers on the figure refer to the numbers in the text.

1 Adverse reaction to food is a pruritic condition.
   • Food trials should be performed when evidence of pruritus has been demonstrated
   • This may be challenging in the cat
   • Adverse reaction to food may be complicated by other pruritic disease or second-ary flare factors

2 Coat brushings and skin scrapes are mandatory before investigating adverse cuta-neous reaction to food.

3, 4 Ectoparasitic disease must be considered before starting a food trial.
   • Adequate flea control is essential both before and during the food trial
   • Scabies should be considered whenever history and clinical signs are consistent
   • Sarcoptes is often not demonstrated on skin scrapes
   • IgG serology is approximately 90% specific and sensitive
   • Trial treatment for scabies should be considered

5 Discuss feasibility of the food trial with the owners.

Appendix 3 is an example of an owner handout which can be used for food trials. A great deal of client support and contact is necessary.
   • The diet must be fed either until the clinical signs resolve or are dramatically improved or until at least 12 weeks have passed
   • No treats, titbits, toys or dietary supplements can be fed during the treatment
   • The contents of any flavoured treatments or gelatine capsules of concomitant treatments should be considered
   • Consider domestic complications of the food trial
   • Young children or older people living in the house who may drop food or be other-wise uncooperative
   • Multi-animal households, especially where ad lib feeding of other pets takes place
   • Untidy teenagers who may leave leftovers around the house
   • Celebrations where there may be various foodstuffs stored and displayed (wed-dings, Christmas, etc.)
   • Cats should ideally be confined to the house. Where this is not possible a trial can still be conducted as the allergen may still be identified, but the owner should be aware of the compromise due to 'outside allergens' ingested

- Scavenging dogs may have to be muzzled on walks or confined
- Neighbours and friends should be warned not to feed the pet
- Home-cooked dietary trials are very laborious and do not suit the modern household. Warn against pre-packed and convenience forms of any protein or carbohydrate sources chosen. Many clients now do not cook for themselves so they are unlikely to cook for their dog or cat
- Many dogs and cats eat leftover takeaway food, making the choice of novel protein and carbohydrate sources extremely difficult
- Many others
- A single treat or mishap means starting the process again.

6 Treat other skin diseases before starting the trial.
- Primary concomitant disease (Chapter 26)
  - Flea bite dermatitis (Chapter 26.1)
  - Other ectoparasitic conditions (Chapter 26.1)
  - Dermatophytosis (Chapter 26.2)
  - Systemic disease
  - Disease secondary to the cause of pruritus (flare factors) (Chapter 27)
  - Bacterial pyoderma (Chapter 27.2)
  - *Malassezia* dermatitis (Chapter 27.2)
  - Secondary keratinisation defects causing greasing and scaling (Chapters 27.3 and 27.4)
  - Flare factors affecting the feet may be especially challenging
  - Localised lesions which may be primary or secondary (Chapter 4)
  - Otitis externa (Chapter 20)
- Clinical signs of ear involvement
- Lesions of the eosinophilic granuloma complex in cats

7 There must be a suitable washout period for all anti-inflammatory treatments before the trial starts. These times are similar to those described for intradermal testing in Table 3.2, but can be simplified as follows:
- Where secondary pyoderma is suspected a course of systemic antibiotics should be given for 2 weeks before the food trial. In severe cases antibiotic treatment can be continued throughout the food trial
- Oral glucocorticoids – 3 weeks
- Long-acting glucocorticoids – at least 3 weeks after duration of action
- Cyclosporin – 3 weeks
- Antihistamines – 1 week
- Topical inflammatory treatments – 1 week
- Aural preparations containing glucocorticoids – 1 week
- Washes and shampoos can be used throughout the trial for patient comfort
- Ectoparasitic treatments should be used throughout the trial
- Avoid other prophylactic treatments during the trial where possible, as flavoured tablets may contain proteins

8 Control flare factors throughout the trial.
- Bacterial pyoderma can be treated with systemic and topical treatments
- *Malassezia* dermatitis can be treated with systemic and topical treatments
- Keratinisation defects can be treated with topical treatments

- All systemic treatments may interfere with the food trial and care in the interpretation of the effects of these treatments is essential.

Continued anti-inflammatory treatments may prove necessary to complete the food trial especially if 12 weeks are required. To assess response to the food trial if this is the case, the treatment should be withdrawn every 3 weeks for 1 week. At the end of the food trial the treatment should be withdrawn to assess the result of the food trial.

9 Selection of trial diet.

A home-cooked diet using protein and carbohydrate sources that the pet doesn't usually eat is the gold standard but is challenging with the ever-increasing types of food fed to pets (and their owners) and ever-decreasing client time.

- Careful history taken of existing diet to identify all proteins and carbohydrates which are fed, including scraps and treats
- A novel protein or carbohydrate source is one which is fed less frequently than once a month
- Choose a novel protein source and novel carbohydrate source for dogs
- Choose a novel protein source only for cats
- Home-cooked fresh ingredients only with no additions – dry roast or boiled in water
- No 'quick' varieties can be used (instant mash, quick rice, etc.)
- Wholemeal grains and unpeeled potatoes should be avoided for contamination

Reasons for choosing a commercial hydrolysed diet (it is better to complete a hydrolysed food trial diet than not to complete a home-cooked one) include

- Patient less than 1 year old (18 months in large breeds)
- Unable to identify novel protein or carbohydrate sources
- Owner unable or unwilling to cook to above restrictions
- Palatability of home-cooked diet likely to cause non-compliance
- Owner unable to cope with hungry pet demanding food

10 Maintain contact with owner at least every 3 weeks.

- Check diet
- Check flare factors
- Check for non-compliance
- Encouragement and reassurance
- Monitor withdrawal of anti-inflammatory treatments where necessary
- Total compliance with the food trial for at least 6 weeks. Twelve weeks may be necessary if a definitive diagnosis cannot be reached before

11 The diet may be diagnostic before 12 weeks.

- If dermatological signs have not reduced a diagnosis of adverse reaction to food can probably be excluded at 2 months, but where doubt remains continue for a further 4–6 weeks
- If dermatological signs have resolved or significantly improved at 6 weeks a provisional diagnosis of adverse reaction to food is made

12 Confirm diagnosis by feeding original diet for 2 weeks.

- If signs do not recur, improvement is coincidental and a diagnosis of adverse reaction to food cannot be made
- All original diet items including scraps and treats should be fed

- Feed elimination diet for 2 weeks
- If signs do not resolve a diagnosis of adverse reaction to food cannot be confirmed

13 If clinical signs recur the trial diet should be reintroduced as strictly as before.
To ensure that improvement is not coincidence due to improvement of seasonal or other disease or flare factors. Pruritus usually improves much more quickly on this second occasion, normally within 2–4 weeks.

14 If clinical signs improve a second time, provocation with dietary proteins should be started.
A number of proteins have been associated with cutaneous adverse reaction to food, although no one protein has been shown to cause reactions more frequently. The most commonly used proteins used in dog food should generally be used first, for example:

- Beef
- Milk
- Chicken
- Eggs
- Lamb
- Wheat
- Soya
- Rice
- Fish

Alternatively, where a commercial diet has been used the restricted diet can be fed long term. Clients are increasingly choosing this option, although these diets are generally more expensive and less palatable than most commercial dog food.

15 A diet can now be formulated for the patient.
- Where possible a commercial diet which has none of the allergens identified should be sourced
- If no commercial diet can be sourced a hydrolysed diet can be trialled
- Home-cooked diets can be formulated using protein and carbohydrate sources which have not caused a recurrence of clinical signs, although they are expensive and time-consuming
- Home-cooked diets are often deficient in micronutrients
- If the owner is reluctant to follow steps 13–15, a hydrolysed diet can be trialled

Clinical signs
- Pruritus, generally persistent in the absence of flare factors or concurrent skin disease (see Figure 12.1)
- Variable erythema, hairloss and secondary signs of inflammation
- Clinical signs similar to other signs of hypersensitivity dermatitis
- No evidence to support anecdotes of predominance of facial lesions or poor response to glucocorticoids
- May be associated with gastrointestinal signs

Principles of treatment
Primary treatment
- Avoid the allergen by feeding diets not containing the allergen

- Can be challenging to identify diets which do not contain the allergen as ingredients found in small amounts or as part of additional fats and proteins are not stated on packaging

Supportive treatment (Chapter 27)
- Treat flare factors
  - Yeast infections – topical miconazole/chlorhexidine shampoos
  - Bacterial infections – systemic and topical antibacterial treatments
  - Parasite control
  - Treat other concurrent hypersensitivity dermatitis

Topical treatments (Chapter 29)
- Shampooing always beneficial
- Choice of shampoo based on clinical signs – pruritus, erythema, scale secondary inflammation, flare factors (Chapter 29)
- Gels, ointments and creams rarely indicated
- Steroid sprays may be indicated for localised lesions

12.4   INSECT BITE HYPERSENSITIVITY

Importance
- Relatively uncommon other than occasional localised lesions
- May present as generalised hives (Figure 2.31) or cutaneous anaphylaxis (Figure 2.30)

Diagnosis
- History
- Environment
- Presence of insects
- Clinical signs
- Supportive histopathology, often with predominance of eosinophils in dermal cellular infiltrate

Clinical signs
- Localised raised erythematous pruritic nodules
- Generalised hives
- Papular rash

Principles of treatment
Primary treatment (Chapter 27.1)
- Systemic or topical glucocorticoids

Supportive treatment
- Avoid insect environment
- Insect repellents

Topical treatments (Chapter 29)
- Gels, creams and ointments may be indicated in localised disease
- Glucocorticoid sprays

- Shampooing beneficial where lesions generalised
- Choice of shampoo based on clinical signs (Chapter 29)

12.5 BACTERIAL, FUNGAL AND YEAST HYPERSENSITIVITY

Importance
- Hypersensitivity to antigens in *Staphylococcus*, *Malassezia* and dermatophytes has been identified

Diagnosis
- History
  - Breed predisposition
  - Staphylococcal – GSD and Bull Terrier
  - *Malassezia* – West Highland White Terrier, Bassett Hound
- Clinical signs
- Identification of micro-organism
- Consistent histopathology with micro-organism identified
- Antigen serology
- Response to treatment

Clinical signs
- Pruritus, erythema and signs of secondary inflammation
- Signs associated with micro-organism
  - Papular/pustular rash
  - Hyperpigmentation
  - Odour
  - Greasiness

Principles of treatment
Primary treatment (Chapter 26.3)
- ASIT treatment of choice
- All other treatments aimed at reducing pruritus
  - Prednisolone or methylprednisolone
  - Cyclosporin
  - Herbal supplements
  - Essential fatty acids
  - Antihistamines
  - (Tricyclic antidepressants and leukotrienes have also been used)

Supportive treatment (Chapter 27)
- Treat flare factors
  - Yeast infections – chlorhexidine/miconazole shampoos
  - Bacterial infections – systemic and topical antibacterial treatments
  - Parasite control – predisposed to flea bite dermatitis
- Dietary supplementation may be beneficial

Hypersensitivity Dermatitis

Rare disorders which may be caused by hypersensitivity reactions

- 'Hormonal hypersensitivity' (see endocrine disease in Chapter 14)

- Endoparasite hypersensitivity has been reported, but there is little or no supporting evidence

Idiopathic pruritus

- In a number of cases a diagnosis of hypersensitivity dermatitis will not be reached despite consistent history and clinical signs
- As the aetiopathogeneses of the hypersensitivity disorders is not fully understood it is likely that a diagnosis will be reached in more of these cases in the future
- It is important that this 'diagnosis' is only made following rigorous diagnostic investigations as management is usually challenging and based on long-term drug control

Principles of treatment
Primary treatment
- Treat pruritus (Chapter 26.1)

Supportive treatments
- Treat flare factors (Chapter 27)
  ○ Yeast infections
  ○ Bacterial infections
  ○ Thorough and repeated parasite control is essential
  ○ Regular review of differential diagnoses
- Dietary supplementation may be beneficial

Topical treatments (Chapter 29)
- Shampooing is always beneficial
- Choice of shampoo based on clinical signs – pruritus, erythema, scale, secondary inflammatory change, flare factors

Chapter 13

Management of Immune-Mediated Disease

Many dermatological diseases whose exact aetiopathogenesis have not been fully elucidated have an immune-mediated component. This description often appears on laboratory reports. With time, some of these diseases will be recategorised and some will be relegated to clinical signs and reaction patterns rather than diagnoses.

13.1   TYPES OF IMMUNE-MEDIATED DISEASE

Diseases caused by immune defects and immunosuppression
- Inherited defects
- Localised specific immune defects, e.g. demodicosis (Chapter 10)

Diseases causing immunosuppression
- Hyperadrenocorticism (Chapter 14)
- Neoplastic disease (Chapter 16)

Diseases caused by abnormal responses to foreign proteins
- Hypersensitivity dermatitis (see Chapter 12)
- Cutaneous adverse reaction to drugs

Diseases caused by abnormal reactions to self-proteins – 'autoimmune disease'
- Diseases where an external trigger factor results in immunological tissue damage
- Autoimmune disease

Increasingly it is found that most of these diseases are immune mediated and that purely intrinsic autoimmune disease is rare, although there are many predisposing factors which point at some intrinsic triggers

This chapter describes the more common diseases caused by abnormal reactions to self-proteins, but includes cutaneous adverse reactions to drugs as the histopathological changes and clinical appearance are often very similar to autoimmune disease.

13.2   THE MANAGEMENT OF IMMUNE-MEDIATED DISEASE

The management of immune-mediated disease is outlined in Figure 13.1. The numbers on the figure refer to the numbers in the text.

1   Reaction pattern
   Clinical signs. The clinical signs may be very helpful in the diagnosis of some immune-mediated skin disease, for example, the often bilaterally symmetrical

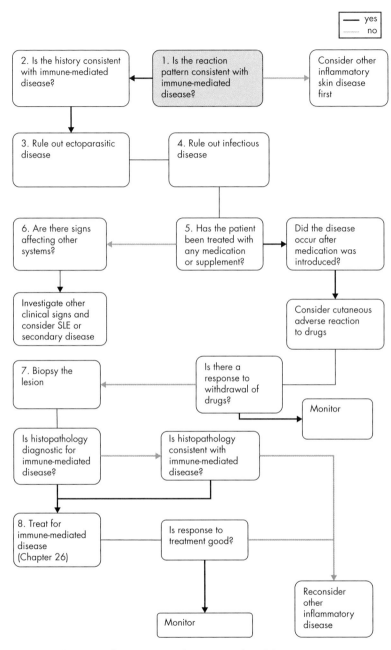

yes
no

2. Is the history consistent with immune-mediated disease?

1. Is the reaction pattern consistent with immune-mediated disease?

Consider other inflammatory skin disease first

3. Rule out ectoparasitic disease

4. Rule out infectious disease

6. Are there signs affecting other systems?

5. Has the patient been treated with any medication or supplement?

Did the disease occur after medication was introduced?

Investigate other clinical signs and consider SLE or secondary disease

Consider cutaneous adverse reaction to drugs

7. Biopsy the lesion

Is there a response to withdrawal of drugs?

Monitor

Is histopathology diagnostic for immune-mediated disease?

Is histopathology consistent with immune-mediated disease?

8. Treat for immune-mediated disease (Chapter 26)

Is response to treatment good?

Reconsider other inflammatory disease

Monitor

Management of Immune-Mediated Disease

Figure 13.1   Flow chart of management of immune-mediated disease.

scaling pattern often seen in pemphigus foliaceus or nasal lesion in discoid lupus erythematosus.

Cytology. Where there are any intact pustules, bullae or vesicles the contents may be helpful in reaching a diagnosis. In immune-mediated disease these lesions may contain healthy neutrophils in all stages of development and acanthocytes may be seen. In contrast in infectious pustules, toxic neutrophils and bacteria are usually seen (Figures 7.3, 7.4). However, in open lesions toxic neutrophils and bacteria are often seen as a secondary feature and experience in taking cytology samples and their examination improves results.

Histopathology. On occasion immune-mediated disease is not suspected until biopsy when histopathological signs consistent with immune-mediated disease are reported. Several reaction patterns may be seen.

If this occurs investigation of immune-mediated disease should be initiated rather than treatment as other diseases may also cause these many of these signs.

2 History

Immune-mediated disease is most common in young and middle-aged females.

Certain breeds are predisposed, e.g. collies.

A careful history should always be taken where immune disease is suspected:
- Identify possible cutaneous adverse reaction to drugs
- Identify trigger factors in drugs, food, environment

Trigger factors for immune-mediated disease are increasingly being identified:
- Drugs
- Feed additives and dyes
- Infectious disease

3 Ectoparasitic disease

Ectoparasitism is an important differential in immune-mediated disease. Immune-mediated disease may result in mild inflammatory change and scaling as also seen in demodicosis, cheyletiellosis and irritation due to lice.

The severe erythematous, pruritic dermatitis seen in scabies can be similar to that seen in some immune-mediated disease.

4 Infectious disease

Systemic infectious disease is a possible trigger factor for immune-mediated disease.

Dermatophytosis should be ruled out as a cause of scaling disease before investigating immune-mediated disease, especially in cats.

Distemper hyperkeratosis can resemble pemphigus foliaceus in the dog.

5 Cutaneous adverse reaction to drugs

Provocation with the suspected medication should never be used as a diagnostic tool.

6 Other clinical signs

The presence of clinical signs of other organ systems or debility may indicate the presence of multisystemic immune-mediated disease such as systemic lupus erythematosus and this should be investigated further.

However, the severe inflammatory changes seen in immune-mediated disease often result in pain, discomfort and disability.

The lesions of skin immune-mediated disease may also become secondarily infected resulting in signs of toxaemia.

7 Histopathological changes
Intact vesicles and bullae containing inflammatory cells and acanthocytes may be diagnostic for immune-mediated disease.

More frequently reaction patterns which are strongly consistent with immune-mediated disease when considered with history and clinical signs may be used for diagnosis.
- Separation of epidermal cell layers
- Interface dermatitis
- Erythema multiforme

A diagnosis of immune-mediated disease is not often ruled out on histopathology alone, unless a definitive diagnosis of another disease is made.

Examples of diseases where there is a strong clinical suspicion of immune-mediated disease and biopsy is essential in making a definitive diagnosis are:
- Sebaceous adenitis
- Necrotic migratory erythema
- Epitheliotrophic lymphoma

8 Principles of treatment
Specific treatment protocols are detailed in Chapter 26. The general principles of treatment of immune-mediated disease are similar, but care should be taken to use less aggressive treatments with less risk of side-effects in more benign diseases and mild forms of the disease.

Primary treatment
- Identify and remove trigger factors where possible
- Investigate disease affecting other organ systems
- Immunosuppressive treatment based on glucocorticoids and other immunomodulating drugs

Supporting treatment
- Pain relief should be considered
- Treat secondary infectious disease

Topical treatment
- Shampooing always beneficial when not too painful
  - Treat secondary infectious disease
  - Remove scale and debris
  - Increase patient comfort
  - Improve absorption of topical treatments
- Topical treatments alone of localised lesions preferable to avoid unnecessary drug side-effects

Management of Immune-Mediated Disease

13.3 SPECIFIC DISEASES

Pemphigus foliaceus (Figures 13.2–13.4)
Importance
- Most common immune-mediated disease
- Trigger factors commonly identified
- Common in cats
- May regress spontaneously

History
- Young and middle-aged females predisposed in spontaneous cases
- Breed predisposition for collie type dogs
- Variable clinical signs, occasionally intermittent at start

Clinical signs
- Feet face head paws predisposed
- May see intact pustules
- Most commonly seen as a scaling dermatosis, often bilaterally symmetrical

Diagnosis
- History
- Clinical signs
- Diagnostic or supportive histopathology

Treatment
- Identify and remove trigger factors
- May regress spontaneously
- May require lifelong immunosuppressive therapy

Prognosis
- Guarded
- Resolution may occur after 6 weeks to 6 months of treatment

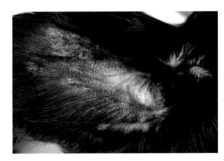

Figure 13.2 Pinnal lesions in pemphigus foliaceus.

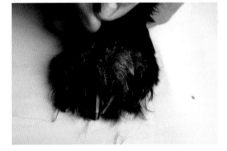

Figure 13.3 Foot lesions in pemphigus foliaceus.

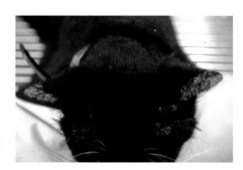

Figure 13.4 Bilaterally symmetrical facial scaling lesions in pemphigus foliaceus.

Cutaneous adverse reaction to drugs

Importance
- Can occur with any drug and food dyes
- Can appear clinically similar to pemphigus foliaceus

History
- Signs may occur in a breed not normally predisposed to immune-mediated disease
- No temporal link between start or cessation of medication and clinical signs
- History of medication may be obscure

Clinical signs
- Can be very variable, similar to many immune-mediated diseases
  - Pemphigus foliaceus like
  - Erythema and pruritus common
  - Variable distribution of lesions

Diagnosis
- History and consistent clinical signs
- Supportive histopathology
  - Pemphigus foliaceus like
  - Interface dermatitis
  - Erythema multiforme
- Lack of temporal association can make diagnosis challenging
- Provocation should not be used as an aid to diagnosis

Prognosis
- Guarded if trigger factor cannot be identified
- Prognosis remains somewhat guarded as time to resolution cannot be predicted

Treatment
Principles of treatment
- Identify and remove trigger
- Removal of trigger alone is rarely sufficient as inflammatory change is severe enough to be self-perpetuating

Primary treatment
- Immunosuppressive systemic treatment for 4–6 weeks initially
- Longer treatment or permanent required in most cases

Supportive treatment
- Nutritional support

Topical treatment
- Always beneficial if patient discomfort allows
- Selection of shampoo should be based on predominant clinical signs (see Chapter 29)

Systemic lupus erythematosus

Importance
- Rare multisystemic immune-mediated disease
- Diagnosis can be challenging

History
- Multifactorial
- Young to middle-aged females predisposed
- Can be confusing

Clinical signs
- Very varied
- Skin lesions are very variable
- Involvement of other systems should raise suspicion in persistent inflammatory disease

Diagnosis
- History and clinical signs
- Positive ANA test
- Supportive histopathology, rarely diagnostic

Prognosis
- Very guarded

Principles of treatment
- Treat all organ systems involved
- Lifelong immunosuppressive therapy usually required

Supportive treatment
- Regular review of clinical signs of multisystemic disease
- Control secondary flare factors

Topical treatment
- Shampooing beneficial if not too uncomfortable for patient
- Choice of shampoo based on clinical signs prevalent

Discoid lupus erythematosus

Importance
- Relatively common
- Usually benign and localised
- Usually responsive to treatment
- Sunlight exacerbates clinical signs

History
- Usually localised to dorsal nose
- Often intermittent initially
- Summer incidence or worsening

Clinical signs
- Very variable from mild scaling to ulceration and bleeding

Diagnosis
- History and clinical signs
- Supportive histopathology, rarely diagnostic

Prognosis
- Good, although intermittent long-term treatment usually required

Principles of treatment
- Do no harm, this is usually a benign disease that generally does not warrant the risk of side-effects from the use of systemic drugs

Primary treatment
- Topical anti-inflammatory treatment is usually sufficient
- Sunscreens should be used when going outside even in winter
- Systemic immunosuppressive treatment only necessary in more severe cases resistant to treatment

Supportive treatment
- Vaseline to prevent cracking of nasal planum

Topical treatment
- See Chapter 29

Lupoid onychodystrophy

Importance
- Relatively common disease of the nail beds
- Usually a diagnosis of elimination (see Figure 18.14)

History
- Slow onset recurrent nail loss, often thought to be due to trauma initially
- Middle-aged dogs

Clinical signs
- Often associated with lameness
- Milder cases – nail shedding
- More severe cases, bleeding and purulent discharge with local lymphadenopathy
- Usually affects most nails

Diagnosis
- History can be misleading, but multiple nail loss
- Eliminate infectious and traumatic causes
- Clinical signs
- Supportive histopathology. Either amputation of third phalanx and submission of whole sample, or longitudinal section taken through dorsal P2 and P3, but technically challenging

Prognosis
- Guarded, may be persistent and recurrent

Principles of treatment
- Do no harm in mild cases as this is a benign disease

Primary treatment
- May respond to topical treatment combined with nutritional support
- More severe cases require immunomodulating systemic treatments

Supportive treatment
- Nutritional support with vitamin E, zinc and essential fatty acids with cofactors may be beneficial
- Consider pain relief in severe cases and where lameness is present
- Consider protective boots for walks
- Treat secondary bacterial and fungal paronychias

Topical treatment
- Always beneficial
- Soaks
  - Increase patient comfort
  - Remove contaminants, debris and inflammatory exudates
  - Aid in the treatment and prevention of secondary bacterial and fungal paronychia

Erythema multiforme (Figure 13.5)
Importance
- A reaction pattern rather than a diagnosis
- Has been associated with other immune-mediated disease, cutaneous adverse reaction to food and drugs

History
- Acute or chronic onset
- May be a history of medication or infectious or metabolic disease

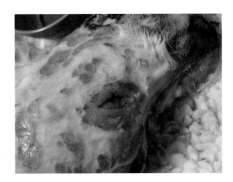

Figure 13.5 Severe lesions of erythema multiforme.

Clinical signs
- Somewhat variable, but erythematous localised spreading lesions
- Variable pruritus or discomfort

Diagnosis
- Identify underlying cause
- Histopathology is consistent finding

Prognosis
- Dependent on underlying cause

Principles of treatment
Primary treatment
- Treat according to the severity of the clinical signs. In some cases no treatment is necessary and no harm should be done in benign cases

Supportive treatment (Chapter 27)
- Aimed at improving patient comfort
- Glucocorticoids and systemic antibacterials may be necessary in severe cases

Topical treatment (Chapter 29)
- Shampoos and washes may be indicated in some cases

Vasculitis
Importance
- The result of an immunological event rather than a diagnosis in most cases
- Relatively uncommon
- May be caused by infection or reaction to drug

History
- Variable depending on underlying cause

Clinical signs
- Often very varied apart from specific disease such as cold agglutinin disease
- Usually localised but may be multisystemic

Diagnosis
- Histopathology

Prognosis
- Generally guarded

Principles of treatment
- Identify underlying cause and remove or correct
- Anti-inflammatory doses of glucocorticoids and other immunomodulating drugs

Rare immune-mediated disease
- Uveodermatologic syndrome (Vogt–Koyanagi syndrome). Presentation with ophthalmic signs is more common than with dermatological signs
- Other forms of pemphigus
- Bullous pemphigoid

Chapter 14
Endocrine Disease

All endocrine disease has the potential to affect the skin due to reduced nutrition to the skin, changes in blood supply and general debility. This chapter is mainly restricted to common endocrine diseases where primary skin signs occur.

14.1   HYPERADRENOCORTICISM

Hyperadrenocorticism (HAC) is a naturally occurring or iatrogenic disease affecting glucocorticoid levels in the dog. HAC is probably the most common endocrine disorder encountered in first opinion practice, but diagnosis and management of these cases remain challenging.

Four forms of the disease occur:
1   Pituitary-dependent HAC (PDHAC)
   a. Caused by a small hormonally active tumour in the pituitary gland
   b. The most common form in most breeds
   c. Controllable but not curable with medication
2   Adrenal-dependent HAC (ADHAC)
   a. Usually caused by adrenal tumour
   b. Can be caused by idiopathic adrenal hyperplasia
   c. Tumours may be benign or malignant and may spread locally
   d. Surgery is the treatment of choice for tumours, though some cases are inoperable due to spread of the tumour.
3   Ectopic active adrenal tissue
   a. Common in man
   b. Few reports in dogs and cats
4   Iatrogenic HAC
   a. Caused by the injudicious use of glucocorticoids
   b. Usually reversible with gradual withdrawal of glucocorticoids

Management of HAC
HAC is probably the most common endocrine disorder encountered in first opinion practice. Figure 14.1 outlines the management of endocrine disease. The numbers in the text refer to the numbers on the figure.

1 History and clinical signs
The history and clinical signs can be extremely varied, but the most common presenting signs are:

• Breed
   ◦ Many breeds predisposed
   ◦ Boxer

Endocrine Disease

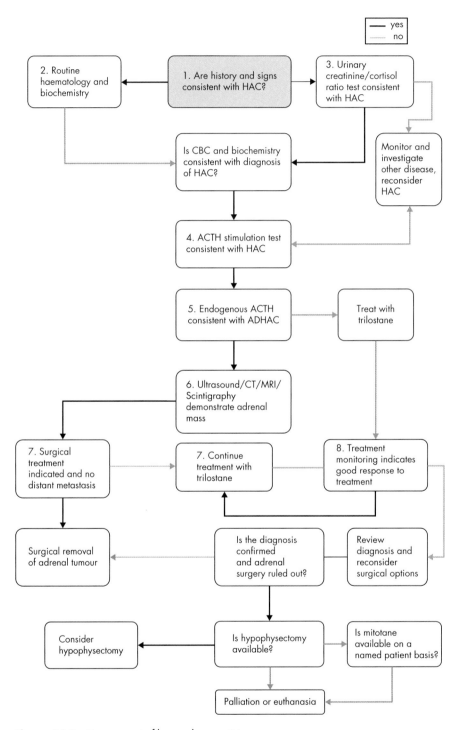

Figure 14.1   Management of hyperadrenocorticism.

- ◦ Poodle
- ◦ Yorkshire Terrier
- ◦ Scottish Terrier
- ◦ Other
- Female more than male
- Middle-aged dogs, unusual to occur younger
- Variable onset, may be mild recurrent before progressive signs develop. May present acutely, occasionally with a single clinical sign
- Polydypsia and polyuria (differentiate from urinary frequency, although cystitis can be a presenting sign)
- Muscle wastage resulting in changing body shape
  - ◦ Prominent occipital crest
  - ◦ Pot belly
  - ◦ Under muscled appearance to legs
- Variation in appetite
- Cutaneous clinical signs (Figure 14.2)
  - ◦ Calcinosis cutis
  - ◦ Skin thinning with prominent cutaneous vessels
  - ◦ Comedones
  - ◦ Recurrent pyoderma
  - ◦ Flank alopecia
  - ◦ Loss of skin elasticity

2 Routine haematology and biochemistry is useful

Haematology may be unremarkable in early disease.

- Leukocytosis, neutrophilia, lymphopaenia and eosinopaenia are all features, especially of chronic HAC
- Biochemistry
- Raised alkaline phosphatase, ALT (isoenzyme in dogs), cholesterol and glucose (cases of diabetes mellitus that are hard to stabilise or on high doses of insulin should be investigated for HAC)

3 Urinary creatinine/cortisol tests

May be useful in ruling out HAC. Urine samples are taken early in the morning on days 1 and 2, then on the third morning before and after administration of ACTH. The test is very sensitive to operator error and stressed patients; testing should be done at home.

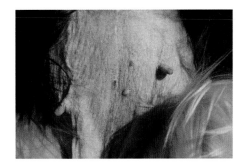

Figure 14.2 Ventral cutaneous lesions of hyperadrenocorticism, comedones, skin thinning, hairloss and reduced elasticity.

Endocrine Disease

4 Dynamic cortisol testing

- Most reliable tests but still many false negatives or positives
- ACTH stimulation test

  Most useful screening test. Diagnostic in 85% cases.

  Take serum sample before and 1 hour after intravenous injection of Synacthen intravenously. Measure cortisol in each sample. Use laboratory ranges for accurate interpretation. Basal samples can be 0–200 nmol/l, samples after stimulation should be 200–600 nmol/l.
- Low dose dexamethasone test

  Take serum sample before and 3 and 8 hours after intravenous injection of 0.01 mg/kg of dexamethasone. Use laboratory ranges for accurate interpretation. Affected dogs do not show suppression of cortisol levels at 3 and 8 hours but normal dogs do.
- High dose dexamethasone test

  More sensitive test, diagnoses more than 95% cases.

  Take serum sample before and 3 and 8 hours after intravenous injection of 0.1 mg/kg of dexamethasone. Use laboratory ranges for accurate interpretation. Normal dogs show suppression at 3 and 8 hours, dogs with pituitary dependent HAC show suppression at 8 hours but not at 3 hours. Dogs with adrenal origin HAC do not suppress at 3 or 8 hours.

Dexamethasone testing has a greater predictive value than ACTH stimulation test but is more sensitive to patient and operator factors and so tends to be of less practical use in practice than ACTH stimulation test combined with endogenous ACTH assay.

5 Endogenous ACTH assay

Very reliable in the diagnosis of HAC and differentiation of PDHAC from ADHAC. High levels of ACTH indicate PDHAC, low levels indicate ADHAC. Contact the investigating laboratory to arrange for frozen transport before taking the sample (see Table 3.3).

6 Imaging

- Radiography often fails to reveal adrenal tumours but may reveal calcification of airways and other calcium deposition and so provide supportive evidence for HAC
- Adrenal tumours can be demonstrated by experienced ultrasonographers
- MRI, CT and scintigraphy can also be used in diagnosis

7 Principles of treatment

Primary treatment

- Adrenal tumours should be removed where possible
- Hypophysectomy is not available in most countries
- Trilostane has a veterinary licence for the control of cortisol levels in pituitary dependent HAC
- opDDD (mitotane) is effective in destroying adrenal tissue in patients who do not respond to trilostane, but is not widely available. Side-effects are common and may be serious. It is an off label use of the drug
- Details of treatment are given in Chapter 26.5

- Prognosis is guarded initially but cases which have a good response to treatment may survive for several years
- Glucocorticoids are contraindicated in the treatment of any other problems from which the patient may suffer

Supportive treatment
- Secondary pyoderma should be treated either with topical or systemic antibacterial agents
- Nutritional support

Topical treatments
- Antibacterial and keratoplastic shampoos
- Topical steroid containing compounds with no systemic absorption may be indicated in lesions of calcinosis cutis causing discomfort

8 Monitoring
- Regular monitoring of treatment using ACTH stimulation test is desirable
- Regular monitoring of thirst and general health by client essential
- Treatment should be tailored to individual patients needs

14.2 HYPOTHYROIDISM

Figure 14.3 outlines the management of hypothyroidism. The numbers in the text refer to the numbers on the figure.

1 History and clinical signs
- Many breeds predisposed
  - Most commonly middle-aged to older dogs
  - Congenital hypothyroidism occurs in some breeds, e.g. Cocker Spaniel
  - Hypothyroidism is very rare in dogs younger than 1 year, except in predisposed breeds, such as the Cocker Spaniel
  - Clinical signs are many and varied. Skin signs may occur in the presence or absence of systemic signs. Skin signs are not always seen
  - Common systemic signs
  - Weight gain or failure to lose weight on a diet (not usually obesity)
  - Lethargy
  - Bradycardia
  - Low rectal temperature
  - Gastrointestinal signs
  - Neurological signs
  - Many others are found occasionally
- A diagnosis of hypothyroidism can rarely be made or excluded on the basis of clinical signs alone
- Common cutaneous signs (Figures 14.4–14.6)
  - Dorsal and flank alopecia
  - Poor hair coat
  - Patchy hairloss ('rat tail')

Endocrine Disease

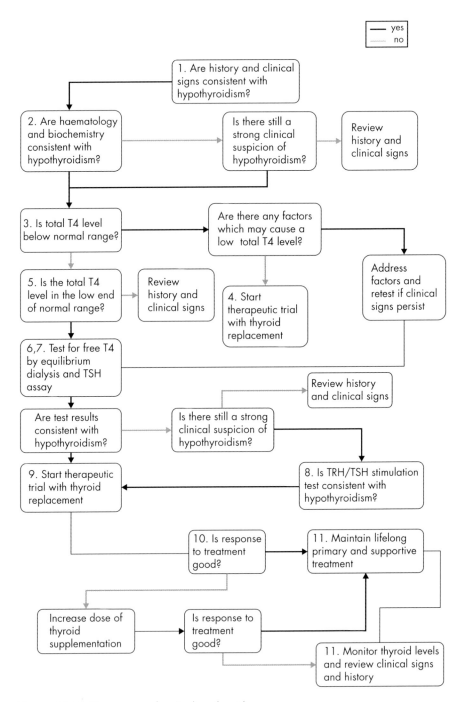

Figure 14.3 Management of canine hypothyroidism.

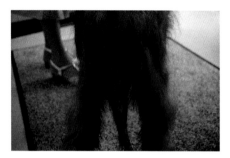

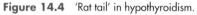

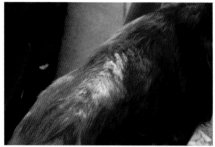

Figure 14.4 'Rat tail' in hypothyroidism.

Figure 14.5 Dorsal hairloss in hypothyroidism.

- ○ Recurrent pyoderma
- ○ Scaling
- ○ Comedone formation
- ○ Hyperpigmentation

2 Routine haematology and biochemistry
- Changes are frequently seen in especially chronic cases of hypothyroidism, but normal blood count and biochemistry does not rule out a diagnosis of hypothyroidism
- Mild normochromic, normocytic anaemia
- Raised cholesterol

3 Total T4 estimation
This is often performed as part of a routine biochemistry screen, and can be useful as a screening test, but is not the test of choice for hypothyroidism.

A number of clinical conditions will cause the total T4 level to be suppressed ('euthyroid' sick syndrome).

A number of commonly used drugs, e.g. prednisolone, potentiated sulphonamides, can cause suppression of T4 levels. Where this is suspected testing should be repeated after withdrawal of these drugs.

Endocrine Disease

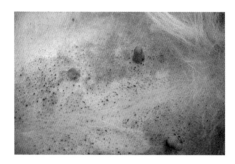

Figure 14.6 Comedones in hypothyroid dog.

4 Therapeutic trial with thyroxin supplementation

Where none of the factors in (3) is an issue a therapeutic trial with levothyronine can be used at this stage and the response to treatment assessed. However, further diagnostic testing is preferable.

5 Low normal total T4 level

A diagnosis of hypothyroidism cannot be ruled out when the total T4 level is in the lower half of the normal range. It is extremely unusual for a diagnosis of hypothyroidism to be made on subsequent testing when the total T4 level is in the upper range.

6 Free T4 by equilibrium dialysis

Free T4 levels are less frequently affected by non-thyroidal illness and equilibrium dialysis is the most accurate measure of free T4. A diagnosis of hypothyroidism can be made with some confidence when free T4 is below the normal range.

7 TSH assay

Raised TSH demonstrates that the feedback mechanism for the production of thyroid hormone is activated and raised TSH levels with low/low normal free T4 can be used together to make a diagnosis of hypothyroidism.

8 TRH/TSH stimulation test

This test can be used to either confirm or exclude a diagnosis of hypothyroidism in cases where there is still a strong clinical suspicion of hypothyroidism and free T4 or TSH assay is inconclusive.

TSH stimulation test is the test of choice but TSH licensed for human in vivo use should be used and is expensive, sometimes being difficult to obtain. Total T4 is estimated before and 4 hours after intravenous injection of TSH. A stimulation of 1.5 times the resting level should be seen in normal dogs.

TRH for human in vivo testing is cheaper and often more easily obtained. However, the stimulation is not as clear. A stimulation of at least 1.25 times the resting level should be seen in normal dogs.

9 Therapeutic trial with levothyronine

A therapeutic trial with levothyronine is started following supportive diagnostic testing.

20 µg/kg once daily is given orally.

A good cutaneous response is usually seen in 6 weeks, although hair regrowth may take up to 12 weeks. Systemic clinical signs may improve more quickly, especially lethargy and exercise tolerance. If clinical response is poor or slow an increased dose of 40 µg/kg can be given for 6 weeks to assess response to treatment.

10 Poor long-term response to treatment

In some cases the requirement for thyroxin is increased. This may be due to exogenous thyroid hormone destruction by autoantibodies to T3 and T4, which can be monitored by measuring autoantibody levels.

11 Principles of treatment

Primary treatment
- Monitor total T4 levels at periodic intervals. Thyroxin levels measured at same time after tablet on each occasion or peak and trough levels can be measured before administration of tablets and 4 hours afterwards
- Maintain primary treatment with levothyronine at therapeutic levels

Supportive treatment
- Regular review of history and clinical signs
- Concomitant disease may be missed if attributed to hypothyroidism
- Skin lesions often not fully responsive
  - Treat secondary pyoderma and *Malassezia* infections
  - Treat scaling, scurfing and greasing

Topical treatment
- Shampooing is always beneficial
- Treat as required for secondary pyoderma
- Regular shampooing for scaling and poor coat condition
- See Chapter 29

14.3 LESS COMMON ENDOCRINE DISEASES WITH A PRIMARY EFFECT ON THE SKIN

Adrenal dysfunction
Testicular tumours
Ovarian dysfunction
Pituitary dwarfism

14.3.1 ADRENAL HYPERPLASIA LIKE SYNDROME (ALOPECIA X, ADRENAL SEX HORMONE IMBALANCE, GROWTH HORMONE RESPONSIVE DERMATOSIS, CASTRATION RESPONSIVE DERMATOSIS)

- Presentation similar to that for 'growth hormone responsive dermatosis'
- Chow and Pomeranian predisposed
- Now thought to be related adrenal sex hormone production effect on growth hormone is secondary to this
- Animal remains clinically well

History
- Young predominantly male animals of predisposed breeds
- Initially coat thinning then total hairloss

Clinical signs (Figures 14.7 and 14.8)
- Progressive hairloss affecting mainly the trunk
- Hyperpigmentation
- No pruritus
- Secondary scaling and pyoderma occasionally occurs

Diagnosis
- History and clinical signs
- Supportive histopathology
- SHAP profile – estimation of cortisol and 17-OH-progesterone before and 1 hour after administration of ACTH intravenously
- 17-OH-progesterone levels are very low in normal dogs, raised in affected dogs, often significantly so after stimulation
- Cortisol levels are normal before and after stimulation

Principles of treatment
Primary treatment
- Melatonin can be used but benefit should be assessed against risks in a disease where effects are cosmetic

Supportive treatment
- Coat and skin condition is often poor so nutritional supplementation may be beneficial

Topical treatments
- Always beneficial for the control of secondary pyoderma and scaling

Prognosis
- Good for general health, poor for hair regrowth

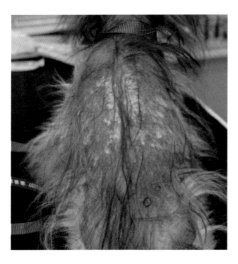

Figure 14.7 Pomeranian with adrenal hyperplasia-like syndrome.

Endocrine Disease

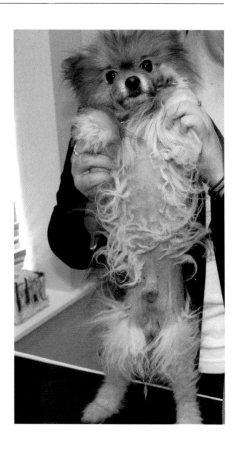

Figure 14.8 Pomeranian with adrenal hyperplasia-like syndrome.

14.3.2 TESTICULAR TUMOURS

- Testicular tumours are more common where there are retained testicles
- Prevalence is highest in abdominally retained testicles
- Increased prevalence both in inguinally retained testicle and also the normally positioned pair of a retained testicle
- Castration of dogs with retained testicles advisable before middle age is reached
- Seminomas and interstitial cell tumours more common, but Sertoli's cell tumour more likely to be hormonally active

History
- Middle-aged males with unilateral or bilaterally retained testicles
- Beware unknown history, assumed removal, etc.
- May be hormonally active or inactive

Clinical signs (Figure 14.9)
- Signs of feminisation
  - Small pendulous prepuce
  - Shrinkage of 'normal' testicle
  - Gynecomastia

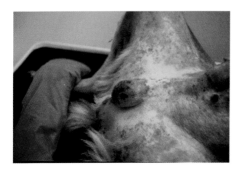

Figure 14.9 Skin changes in testicular tumour.

- Flank and ventral alopecia
- Poor coat condition, scaling secondary pyoderma

Principles of treatment
Primary treatment
- Surgical removal of both testicles

Supportive treatment
- Metastasis search before surgery
- Nutritional support may be beneficial for poor coat condition and scaling
- Antibacterial treatment for secondary pyoderma

Topical treatment
- Contraindicated in the interval between surgery and suture removal
- Always beneficial at other times
- May be indicated for several months
- See Chapter 29

Prognosis
- Good, although some tumours are malignant more than 50% can be removed before local spread or distant metastasis occurs

14.4 COMMON ENDOCRINE DISEASES THAT HAVE A SECONDARY EFFECT ON THE SKIN

14.4.1 FELINE HYPERTHYROIDISM

- Although a common and important condition in the cat, the presenting signs are usually systemic rather than dermatological
- Dermatological signs are secondary and related to debility and reduced grooming

Diagnosis
- History and clinical signs, usually a disease of middle-aged and older cats
- Weight loss usually noted as first sign by owner
- Change in temperament

- Unkempt appearance
- Heart rate over 200 bpm highly suspicious
- Raised total thyroxin levels on blood biochemistry

Management
- Primary disease should be addressed (see Chapter 26)
- Treatment of poor hair coat and scaling will increase patient comfort (see Chapters 27, 29)

14.4.2   DIABETIC DERMATOSIS

- Although a common and important condition in the dog and cat, patients are usually presented with systemic signs initially
- Occasionally a patient may present with only recurrent pyoderma
- Other changes include poor hair coat and scaling
- Secondary pyoderma, *Malassezia* and fungal infections are important
- Conversely poorly responsive pyoderma, *Malassezia* dermatitis and dermatophytosis should be screened for diabetes mellitus

Diagnosis
- History and clinical signs
  - Some breeds predisposed – poodle, cocker spaniel
  - Common in middle aged
  - Obesity predisposes
  - Entire females predisposed
  - Repeatable raised fasting blood glucose levels
  - Glycosuria
  - Dermatological signs in predisposed patients

Management
- Protocols for the primary treatment and control of diabetes mellitus are found in all standard medicine texts and are not included in this book
- Secondary dermatological problems should be treated according to the presenting clinical signs (see Chapters 27, 29)

14.5   RARE ENDOCRINE PROBLEMS

- Sex hormone dysfunction in entire and neutered animals
- Hyperoestrogenism temporal relationship to oestrous cycle
- Pituitary dwarfism
- Hypothyroidism in the cat – there is one report of naturally occurring acquired hypothyroidism
- HAC in the cat
- HAC in the guinea pig
- Acromegaly in the dog and cat

Non-endocrine alopecias are described in Chapter 15.

Endocrine Disease

Chapter 15

Disorders of the Pilosebaceous Unit (Hair Follicle Disorders)

Endocrine disorders resulting in damage to the pilosebaceous unit are described in Chapter 14.

Secondary hair follicle disorders are more common than primary ones. Table 15.1 shows the more common causes of hair follicle disorders.

Diagnosis
Hair follicle dysplasias are usually suspected on the basis of history and clinical signs, but diagnosis is usually confirmed on histopathology of biopsy specimens.

15.1 PRIMARY HAIR FOLLICLE DYSPLASIAS

15.1.1 HAIRLESS BREEDS

- Bred for hair follicle dysplasia
- Mexican hairless dog
- Chinese crested dog
- Sphinx cat
- Cornish and Devon Rex cats
- May result in severe keratinisation disorders. Palliative treatment only
- See Chapters 27, 29

15.1.2 COLOUR DILUTION ALOPECIA (COLOUR MUTANT ALOPECIA)

- Affects the dilute hair coat of affected dogs
- Seen in blue Dobermanns, Yorkshire Terriers, German Shepherds, etc. Also seen in fawn coats of tan breeds (Figure 15.1)

Table 15.1 Causes of pilosebaceous (hair follicle) disorders

Primary	Secondary
Hairless and hypotrichotic breeds	Endocrine alopecias
Colour dilution alopecia	Telogen and anagen defluxions
Black hair follicular dysplasia	(Sebaceous adenitis)
Other follicular dysplasias	Inflammatory skin disease
Pattern alopecias	Trauma and burns
(Sebaceous adenitis)	

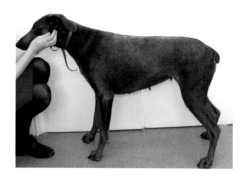

Figure 15.1 Colour dilution alopecia in a Dobermann.

- Was thought to be due to a recessive gene but is also seen in cross breeds demonstrating the dilute coat colour
- Clinical signs of patchy hairloss and secondary scaling and pyoderma may not be seen until 3–4 years of age or older (Figure 15.2), giving 'moth-eaten' appearance
- Head usually spared
- There is no effective treatment of the primary cause
- Treat secondary scaling and pyoderma as necessary (see Chapters 27, 29)

15.1.3 SEBACEOUS ADENITIS

- An immune-mediated reaction aimed specifically at the pilosebaceous unit (hair follicle and sebaceous glands)
- First seen in poodles, now recorded in many breeds
- Strong breed predispositions suggest a genetic cause
- Often bilaterally symmetrical, usually dorsal
- May start at the head and spread backwards or start as patchy hairloss

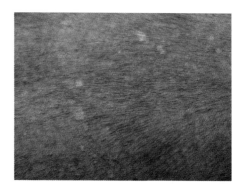

Figure 15.2 Lesions of colour dilution alopecia.

Disorders of the Pilosebaceous Unit (Hair Follicle Disorders)

- Prompt diagnosis and treatment will reduce hair follicle and sebaceous gland destruction and hence reduce hairloss
- Primary treatment is aimed at the inflammatory response. Synthetic retinoids, cyclosporin and glucocorticoids have all been used with some success, all off label (Chapter 26)
- Treatment of secondary scaling, pyoderma and pruritus important (see Chapters 27, 29)
- Warn owners of the likelihood of permanent partial hairloss

15.1.4 OTHER HAIR FOLLICLE DYSPLASIAS

- Black hair follicle dysplasia occurs rarely in the black coats of various breeds such as Dobermanns
- These dysplasias are diagnosed on histopathology, so early biopsy of cases presenting with patchy hairloss, especially in young healthy dogs is essential
- There is no primary treatment, but control of secondary scaling and pyoderma will increase patient comfort (see Chapters 27, 29)

15.1.5 PATTERN ALOPECIAS

- These occur in a number of breeds including the Dachshund and Yorkshire Terrier
- There is no primary treatment and they are usually asymptomatic

15.2 SECONDARY HAIR FOLLICLE DYSPLASIAS

15.2.1 ENDOCRINE (SEE CHAPTER 14)

- Occurs in most endocrine diseases, but hair follicle changes may be absent or non-specific
- Hypothyroidism frequently results in specific hair follicle degeneration
- Hyperadrenocorticism and adrenal gland dysplasias may produce less specific changes
- Treatment is aimed at the underlying cause. Full hair growth is often not achieved

15.2.2 ANAGEN AND TELOGEN DEFLUXIONS

- Hairloss resulting from endocrine changes and other factors such as stress
- For example, telogen defluxion in the post-parturient bitch
- There is no specific treatment
- Resolves spontaneously after several weeks
- Palliative measures may increase patient comfort where there is secondary scaling, inflammation or pyoderma (Chapters 27, 29)

15.2.3   INFLAMMATORY SKIN DISEASE

- Hairloss resulting from folliculitis in any inflammatory skin disease
- Treatment is aimed at correcting the underlying cause
- Follicle damage is usually reversible except in very severe cases

15.2.4   TRAUMA AND BURNS

- May result in damage or destruction of the hair follicles
- Where hair follicles are destroyed hairloss will be permanent
- Where the epidermis is destroyed hairloss will be permanent

Disorders of the Pilosebaceous Unit
(Hair Follicle Disorders)

Chapter 16

Neoplastic Skin Disease

This section is a general overview of neoplasia in skin disease. The reader should refer to suitable oncological and surgical texts for more detail on treatment.

Biopsy and histopathological examination is mandatory for all masses. Further advice should be sought from the histopathologist on an individual case basis.

- Primary skin tumours
  - Discrete and solitary masses
  - Multiple or diffuse skin masses
- Secondary skin neoplasia
- Paraneoplastic syndromes

16.1 PRIMARY SKIN MASSES

Figure 16.1 describes the management of primary skin masses. The numbers in the text refer to the numbers on the figure.

1 Discrete solitary masses (except suspected mast cell tumours and mammary masses)

- Removal of all such masses should be advised, except where the clinical condition of the patient precludes this
- Aspiration or impression smear cytology may aid decision making, but negative findings should not be overinterpreted (Chapter 3)
- Where an owner declines mass removal, the size and the character of the mass should be recorded so that a decision for future removal can be made
- Ideally, all masses should be sent for histopathology unless the tumour type can be determined for certainty on gross examination (e.g. some lipomas)
- Where masses are not sent for histopathology they should be kept for future reference

2 Masses in areas where risk of malignancy is increased should be staged and treated as if they were potentially malignant

- This includes mammary and perianal, digital and oral masses
- Masses which may prove challenging to remove should be included in this group
- Masses which have features consistent with mast cell tumours should also be included
- Masses on the leg should be carefully evaluated before removal is attempted as closure following removal with adequate margins may prove difficult
- Aspiration or impression smear cytology may aid decision making, but negative findings should not be overinterpreted

3 Clinical assessment

- Further assessment, for example complete blood counts, should be considered
- Perianal and mammary masses

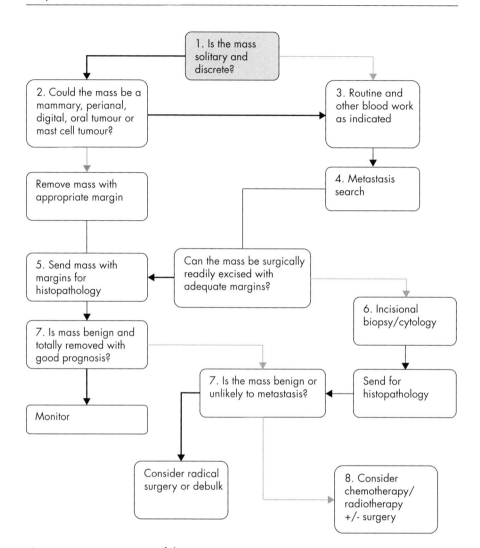

Figure 16.1 Management of skin masses.

- To assist in the identification of the primary site where secondary malignancy is suspected
- Where paraneoplastic syndromes are suspected
- Where metastatic spread is suspected
- Where systemic signs of disease are present

4 Further investigation before mass removal

Where malignancy is suspected a search for metastasis should be carried out before excision of the mass. This most frequently will consist of blood testing and chest radiography, but in some cases more sophisticated techniques may be employed.

5 Where the mass can be readily removed in its entirety this should be done

- Aspiration or impression smear cytology may aid in decision making regarding adequate margins of excision

- Where possible the entire mass and its margins should be submitted for histopathology
- Predisposing factors for recurrence should be addressed, for example, castration of dogs with perianal adenomas
- Ovariohysterectomy of bitches with mammary tumours is recommended, although evidence supports reduced recurrence only in younger bitches

6 Where the mass cannot be removed completely without major surgical reconstruction
- Incisional biopsy following staging is preferable to aspiration or impression smear cytology
- Specific expertise is required for the examination of these samples

7 Benign mass
- Where complete removal of a benign mass with adequate margins has been achieved no further action is generally required, although the owner should be asked to monitor the patient at regular intervals
- Care should be taken with benign masses with a tendency to recur, such as haemangioperiocytoma
- Where a mass is benign or distant metastasis is unlikely
- Where possible the mass should be removed with adequate margins and surgical reconstruction performed
- Where this is not possible palliative debulking of the mass may be carried out if appropriate following discussion with the owner

8 Consider chemotherapy or radiotherapy
- Where the mass is inoperable or where the neoplasm is generalised, specialist expertise regarding chemotherapy or radiotherapy should be sought

Table 16.1 shows the features commonly associated with benign and malignant skin tumours. These features alone should not be relied on in the management of skin tumours, but may be useful for guidance.

Table 16.1 Features commonly associated with benign and malignant skin tumours

Benign skin tumours	Malignant skin tumours
Slow growing	Rapidly growing
Discrete	Local spread
Freely mobile	Skin or deep attachment
Smooth surface	Rough or even surface
Little change in skin surface	Change in pigment or ulceration
Cells resemble tissue of origin	Pleomorphism
Low number of mitotic figures	High number of mitotic figures
Low tendency to recurrence	High tendency to recurrence
No metastatic spread	High tendency to metastatic spread
Frequently sited on trunk	Increased incidence at extremities
Tend to grow outwards	Tend to grow inwards and laterally

For example,

- Benign histiocytoma has high number of mitotic figures
- Malignant squamous cell carcinoma (SCC) does not frequently metastasise
- Cutaneous mast cell tumour may vary considerably in all features and malignancy
- Malignant transformation of benign tumour may occur
- Recurrence of benign perianal adenoma in entire males
- Recurrence of haemangiopericytoma

Mammary tumours of similar appearance (Figure 16.2) can be benign, malignant or mixed.

Mast cell tumours require careful investigation as it is not possible to predict malignancy from appearance.

16.2 COMMON TYPES OF SKIN NEOPLASIA

16.2.1 MAST CELL TUMOUR

- May be clinically indistinguishable from other types of skin neoplasia
- Behaviour variable from benign to extremely malignant
- May see local swelling and occasional anaphylactic response after handling due to histamine release from mast cells (Table 16.2)

Treatment
- Surgery is treatment of choice
- May be variably responsive to chemotherapy
- Prednisolone may be effective as a palliative measure
- Kinase inhibitors have recently been introduced for treatment

16.2.2 SQUAMOUS CELL CARCINOMA (FIGURE 16.3)

- Common in the cat, occurs in other species
- Ear tip and nose are predilection sites

Neoplastic Skin Disease

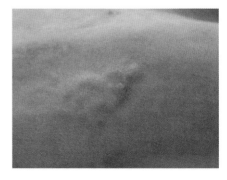

Figure 16.2 Mammary tumour in a bitch.

Table 16.2 Common types of skin neoplasia

Benign tumours	Malignant tumours
Mast cell tumour	Mast cell tumour
Basal cell tumour	Squamous cell carcinoma
Melanoma	Melanoma
Histiocytoma (Langerhans cell tumour)	Epitheliotrophic lymphoma
Adnexal tumours	

Treatment
- Pinnal amputation is generally curative in ear tip SCC
- Nasal tumours can be removed with constructive surgery
- Poorly responsive to chemotherapy

16.2.3   MELANOMA

- May be benign or malignant
- Toe and oral location predisposes to malignancy
- Often slow to metastasise

Treatment
- Surgery is treatment of choice
- Poorly responsive to chemotherapy
- Responsive to radiotherapy where available

16.2.4   SKIN 'LUMPS AND BUMPS'

- Common in middle-aged and older animals, especially dogs
- Skin masses are more likely to be malignant in cats than dogs
- Each mass should be evaluated on an individual basis
- Histopathology should be performed on entire masses removed with the skin margin intact

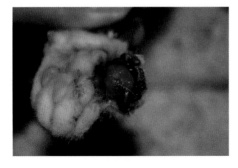

Figure 16.3   SCC on the toe of a cat.

Neoplastic Skin Disease

16.2.5   PRECANCEROUS CHANGES

Outgrowths of keratin ('cutaneous horns') have been reported to be associated with precancerous change which may undergo malignant transformation (Figure 16.4).

16.3   GENERALISED SKIN NEOPLASIA

16.3.1   MULTIPLE MAST CELL TUMOUR (FIGURE 16.5)

- Usually malignant
- Prognosis very poor

Treatment
- Surgery not usually an option
- May be responsive to chemotherapy
- Poorly responsive to radiotherapy
- Palliation with glucocorticoid treatment may prolong quality of life

16.3.2   EPITHELIOTROPHIC LYMPHOMA (FIGURE 16.6)

Dog/Cat/Hamster
Diagnosis
- History
- No breed predisposition
- Average age 11 years in dog

Clinical signs
- Erythematosus scaling disease, localised → generalised
- Slow progression
- Mucocutaneous crusting and ulcerating disease similar to AI disease

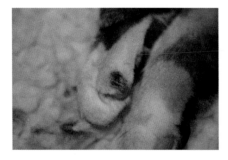

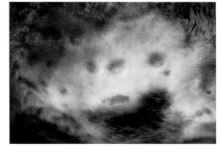

Figure 16.4   Cutaneous horn associated with precancerous change on the toe of a cat.

Figure 16.5   Multiple mast cell tumours on the abdomen of a dog.

Neoplastic Skin Disease

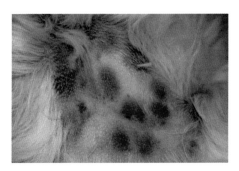

Figure 16.6 Unusual presentation of epitheliotrophic lymphoma in a dog.

- Cats may show discrete scaling alopecic lesions similar to dermatophytosis
- Frequent peripheral lymphadenopathy with systemic illness
- Excision biopsy – histopathology is diagnostic

Treatment
- Palliation with glucocorticoids and shampoos
- Cyclosporin and retinoids have been used with limited success in dogs and cats
- Mustard gas has been suggested, but serious health and safety issues and little success reported
- Lomustine has recently been used in a number of cases and has been tolerated fairly well. Lomustine is very expensive in the UK
- Interferon used with temporary success in one cat

Prognosis
- Very guarded although palliation may be successful for several months
- Euthanasia usually due to secondary inflammatory disease, pyoderma and patient discomfort and debility

16.4 METASTATIC SKIN NEOPLASIA

- A number of primary tumours may metastasise to the skin
- Diagnosis is based on history, clinical signs and histopathological examination of multiple skin biopsies
- Representative samples are usually diagnostic, but care should be taken in sampling as the margin between neoplastic tissue and surrounding inflammation may be diffuse
- Multiple sampling will reduce the risk of missing neoplastic tissue
- Prognosis is usually grave

16.5 PARANEOPLASTIC SYNDROMES

- Hyperadrenocorticism (Chapter 14)
- Hyperthyroidism in the cat (Chapter 14)
- Superficial necrolytic dermatitis

Neoplastic Skin Disease

- Exfoliative dermatitis in thymoma – rare
- Feminising syndromes and alopecia in testicular neoplasia (see Chapter 14)
- Alopecia and gynaecomastia in ovarian neoplasia

16.5.1 SUPERFICIAL NECROLYTIC DERMATITIS (HEPATOCUTANEOUS SYNDROME, METABOLIC EPIDERMAL NECROSIS, NECROLYTIC MIGRATORY ERYTHEMA)

- Uncommon in the dog rare in the cat, reported in the rabbit
- Associated with pancreatic and hepatic neoplasia
- Bilaterally symmetrical scaling condition of gradual onset may precede any other clinical sign of the systemic neoplasia
- Footpad, face, perianal and prepuce most frequently affected
- Prognosis grave, though course of disease may be prolonged and patient may remain clinically well for several months
- Partially responsive to palliative treatments (see Chapters 27 and 29)

Chapter 17
Other Skin Diseases

17.1 METABOLIC DISEASE

17.1.1 DIABETIC DERMATOSIS

See Chapter 14.

In some cases of diabetes mellitus the hair coat may become thin and scaling. Palliative measures (see Chapter 27) will increase patient comfort.

Secondary pyoderma is also common in diabetes mellitus and may be a presenting sign for the disease. Pyoderma is controlled by the use of antibiotics and topical treatments especially shampoos (see Chapter 29).

17.1.2 HYPERADRENOCORTICISM

See Chapter 14.

Patients with hyperadrenocorticism may present with skin thinning, hairloss, scaling, pyoderma or calcinosis cutis, as well as abnormalities of the cutaneous blood vessels. Although these problems may resolve with effective treatment they should be treated symptomatically to increase patient comfort. Calcinosis cutis may result in considerable patient discomfort and pruritus. The use of antibacterial drugs to control secondary pyoderma, shampoos to remove debris and topical anti-inflammatory agents with minimal absorption to reduce the inflammation surrounding the calcium deposits are beneficial (Chapters 27 and 29). Skin fragility and an unkempt coat are often seen in the cat.

17.1.3 HYPOTHYROIDISM

See Chapter 14.

Patients with hypothyroidism may present with hairloss, scaling and secondary pyoderma. The use of antibacterial drugs to control secondary pyoderma and shampoos to remove debris is beneficial (Chapters 27 and 29).

17.1.4 SUPERFICIAL NECROLYTIC DERMATITIS (HEPATO-CUTANEOUS SYNDROME, METABOLIC EPIDERMAL NECROSIS, NECROLYTIC MIGRATORY ERYTHEMA)

See Chapter 16.

May result in scaling hairloss, pruritus and secondary pyoderma. The use of shampoos to remove debris is beneficial and glucocorticoids are a useful palliative measure (Chapters 27 and 29).

17.1.5 OTHER PARANEOPLASTIC SYNDROMES

These are rare (see Chapter 16).

17.2 NUTRITIONAL DISEASE

17.2.1 MALNUTRITION

Rare, but chronic malnutrition due to systemic disease or neglect may result in hairloss scaling and poor coat condition. Related environmental conditions may also result in pressure sores. The primary cause should be addressed and the diet corrected. Topical treatments will improve coat condition and dietary supplementation with essential fatty acids, zinc and other cofactors may increase speed of response and cosmetic condition.

17.2.2 OBESITY

- Common
- Often associated with inappropriate diet leading to scaling and poor coat condition
- May result in reduced grooming in cats leading to scaling, greasiness and fur matting
- Major cause of intertriginous dermatitis in dogs

Treatment
- Address the primary cause with appropriate restricted diet
- Topical treatment of clinical signs, especially bathing of affected areas
- Topical glucocorticoids may be indicated; systemic antibacterial treatment is rarely necessary

17.2.3 ZINC RESPONSIVE DERMATOSIS

- Now uncommon due to loading of commercial diets with zinc
- May still occur in dogs fed poor generic diets with high cereal contents as phytates in cereals compete with zinc for intestinal absorption
- Diagnosis made on history of diet and clinical signs (bilaterally symmetrical scaling affecting the face). Diagnosis confirmed on histopathological examination (parakeratosis)
- Occurs as two syndromes:
  ◦ Genetic in Alaskan malamutes
  ◦ Juvenile form in Labrador retrievers, etc.

Treatment
- Correct diet
- 200 mg zinc sulphate capsules daily for 6 weeks
- Vomiting is common due to gastric irritant effect of zinc sulphate. Give with food or split capsules and spread on food

Other Skin Diseases

17.2.4 VITAMIN A RESPONSIVE DERMATOSIS

- Uncommon problem affecting Cocker Spaniels
- Diagnosis usually made on clinical signs of scaling and histopathological examination. Responds to high doses of vitamin A and supportive treatment for scaling (see Chapters 27 and 29)

17.2.5 VITAMIN AND MINERAL DEFICIENCIES

Rare but may be challenging to diagnose. All patients with chronic dermatoses should be fed good quality commercial diets to correct any underlying deficiencies.

17.3 ENVIRONMENTAL CAUSES

17.3.1 SUNLIGHT RELATED DISEASE

- There is a causal link between squamous cell carcinoma of the pinnae in cats and exposure to sunlight (see Chapter 16). This is often preceded by a scaling erythematous dermatitis
- Sunlight may predispose to other neoplastic disease
- Sunlight may exacerbate some immune-mediated disease, for example, discoid lupus erythematosus
- White coated animals and dogs who sunbathe on their backs may suffer from sunburn

17.3.2 THERMAL AND CHEMICAL BURNS

- Occur occasionally
  - Patients in lateral recumbency on heated pads
  - Dogs and cats may suffer burns to the oral cavity when eating inappropriate substances
  - Plasma cell pododermatitis in cats is often mistaken for burns attributed to walking on hot plates or chemicals
  - Dogs may show multiple pad trauma after running on hot pavements with their jogging owners
- Contact with exhaust pipes during road traffic accident
- Treatment is symptomatic

17.3.3 COLD

- Frost bite is rare
- Cold agglutinin reaction is rare
- Acromelanism demonstrated by some cat breeds may result in a dark patch of hair growing over surgical sites which will resolve at the next moult

17.3.4 HUMIDITY

- Increased humidity adversely affects most skin disease. Increased surface moisture increases microbial flora and in severe circumstances, maceration of the tissue occurs, especially in skin folds
- Examples include:
  - Pyotraumatic dermatitis
  - Lip, tail and facial fold dermatitis (see Chapters 19, 22 and 23)
- Increased humidity may result in bacterial or yeast otitis externa in stenotic ear canals, inflammatory skin disease or where external ear canals become waterlogged during swimming or bathing (see Chapter 20)

17.3.5 PRESSURE SORES

See Chapter 24.

17.3.6 TRAUMA

Wounds, burns, scalds, bites, cat bite abscess and cellulitis

17.4 PSYCHOGENIC DERMATOSES

- Tail chewing
- Foot chewing
- Acral lick dermatitis/furunculosis (see Chapter 24)
- Psychogenic alopecia. This condition has been reported in housed pedigree cats, but is rare. A diagnosis can only be made following a careful investigation of all the physical causes of hairloss in the cat (see Chapter 6). Treatment is based on correcting the underlying husbandry
- These may respond to behaviour altering drugs, but careful investigation of underlying causes and their management should be undertaken before initiating drug therapy and the advice of a behaviourist should be sought before undertaking long-term therapy

17.5 DERMATOSES OF NEUROLOGICAL ORIGIN

- It is important to differentiate these from the inflammatory causes of pruritic skin disease (Chapter 4)
- These are rare
- Hyperaesthesia leading to leg and tail biting
- Acral mutilation syndromes
- Syringomyelia (Chiari like syndrome) in the Cavalier Spaniel resulting in head-shaking

Other Skin Diseases

SECTION 4

ANATOMICALLY LOCALISED SKIN DISEASE

Chapter 18

The Foot

Skin disease can occur either as a condition affecting only the foot or as part of a generalised skin disease. Conditions affecting the foot present particular difficulties due to:

- Specialised anatomy of the foot
  - Claw
  - Footpad
  - Concentrations of sebaceous and sweat glands
  - Intertriginous areas between the toes
- Contamination and trauma due to contact with ground
- Predilection site for some diseases, e.g. pododemodicosis
- Predilection site for licking and chewing
- Similar clinical presentation regardless of underlying cause in many conditions

The specialised structure of the foot, folded skin, thickened tissues with a poor blood supply, and distribution of sebaceous and sweat glands, results in a greater therapeutic challenge in diseases where the foot is involved.

Owners should be warned that longer and more aggressive treatment is often needed and that the prognosis is more guarded than with less specialised areas of skin.

Foot problems can often present major problems in rabbits and rodents due to poor husbandry. Wet and dirty environmental conditions may result in macerated tissues.

Table 18.1 lists skin conditions commonly affecting the foot.

Table 18.2 lists common conditions localised to the foot.

Three anatomical areas of the feet need to be considered separately:
- The claws
- The footpads
- The less specialised skin of the feet

18.1 MANAGEMENT OF CLAW DISEASE

Figure 18.1 outlines the management of nail and claw disease. The numbers in the text refer to the numbers on the figure.

The Foot

Table 18.1 Generalised skin diseases which commonly involve the foot

Dog

Parasites	Demodicosis Scabies Neotrombiculosis Ticks Hookworm dermatitis Pelodera dermatitis	Demodicosis Neotrombiculosis Ticks
Infection	Deep pyoderma/furunculosis Pyoderma (usually secondary) Bacterial paronychia Distemper Papilloma virus *Malassezia* dermatitis Dermatophytosis Other fungal disease Leishmaniosis Rocky Mountain Spotted Fever	Feline leprosy *Malassezia* dermatitis Dermatophytosis
Hypersensitivity	Atopic dermatitis Food intolerance Other Bacterial Contact Drug eruption	Atopic dermatitis Food intolerance Other Bacterial Contact
Keratinisation defects	Primary, e.g. idiopathic and genetic Secondary to underlying causes	Primary, e.g. idiopathic and genetic Secondary to underlying causes
Pigmentary changes	Vitiligo	Vitiligo
Endocrine	Hypothyroidism Hyperadrenocorticism	
Nodular and granulomatous diseases	Neoplasia (see below) Idiopathic granuloma and pyogranuloma	Neoplasia (see below)
Immune mediated	Pemphigus Leishmaniosis Drug reaction Systemic lupus erythematosus Familial canine dermatomyositis	Pemphigus foliaceus Drug reaction Plasma cell pododermatitis
Neoplasia	Many Plasmacytoma, Mast cell Tumour Melanoma Squamous cell carcinoma Metastatic carcinoma	Squamous cell carcinoma, haemangiosarcoma

Paraneoplastic syndromes	Necrolytic migratory erythema Paraneoplastic pemphigus	Necrolytic migratory erythema Paraneoplastic alopecia
Nutritional	Zinc responsive dermatitis Malnutrition	Malnutrition
Miscellaneous	Acral mutilation syndrome Frostbite Epidermolysis bullosa Epidermal dysplasia Ichthyosis Canine uveodermatologic syndrome Vasculitis Cryoglobulinaemia and cryofibrinogenaemia	Pseudopelade

1 Biopsy visible masses, raised or ulcerated lesions

Biopsy of only the nail and surrounding soft tissue does not yield useful results. Two techniques are used:

(a) Amputation of the distal phalanx and submission of this material including the nail and surrounding soft tissues.

or

(b) A dorsal longitudinal section is taken through the nail bed tissues from the level of the distal phalanx, including bony material. This technique is much more demanding, and there is an increased risk of failing to biopsy representative tissue, but the resulting wound is cosmetically more appealing as all the basic structures are preserved.

2 Treat acute cases empirically but monitor carefully

This includes the loss of a single nail, inflammation and infection due to trauma and incidents where the set of nails is lost over a short period of time and there is no repetition of a single nail loss.

- Removal of the nail frequently indicated
- Systemic antibiotic treatment (see Chapter 27.2)
- Topical washes and rinses (see Chapter 29)
- Avoid further damage to the dermis to facilitate normal regrowth of the nail

Investigation of the underlying disease indicated on first presentation:
- Where demodicosis suspected
- In the presence of nodular, ulcerative or bleeding disease
- Change in pigmentation
- Recurrence of paronychia or nail bed crumbling or breaking
- Where immune-mediated disease is suspected

The Foot

Table 18.2 Conditions localised to the foot

	Footpad	Nail and claw	Skin of foot
Parasitic	Hookworm dermatitis	No common examples	Hookworm dermatitis Scabies Demodicosis Trombiculosis
Infection	Distemper	Bacterial, yeast and fungal paronychia FeLV dermatitis related paronychia Blastomycosis Sporotrichosis Cryptococcosis	Deep pyoderma/ furunculosis Papilloma virus *Malassezia* dermatitis Dermatophytosis
Keratinisation defects	Nasodigital hyperkeratosis Familial pad keratosis	No common examples	No common examples
Immune mediated	Pemphigus complex Plasma cell pododermatitis	Lupoid onychodystrophy Pemphigus complex	Pemphigus complex
Neoplasia	No common examples	Melanoma Squamous cell carcinoma Other	Melanoma Squamous cell carcinoma Haemangiosarcoma Other
Trauma	Cuts and lacerations Corns Blisters from friction and heat	Nail injury following RTA, etc.	Foot chewing
Foreign bodies	Glass, thorns, etc.	No common examples	Grass seeds, etc.
Miscellaneous	Proliferative disorder of footpad Disorder of footpads in GSD	No common examples	Foot chewing as a habit or displacement activity

3 Where foot disease occurs as part of a more generalised disease investigate as for generalised skin disease (see Sections 2 and 3)

4 Where only one toe is affected neoplasia should be ruled out at an early stage

Take skin scrapes for *Demodex* spp. bearing in mind that the mite can be hard to find on the feet. Biopsies should assist in diagnosis of this condition. Usually associated with more generalised pododermatitis.

Take samples for fungal culture. Dermatophytosis restricted to the toes is relatively common. Removed toe nails can be used for fungal culture.

Bacterial culture is less likely to be rewarding as the area is likely to be contaminated and intact pustules are rare.

Biopsy the toe. Amputation of the third phalanx with associated soft tissue structures should be performed; higher amputation may be necessary.

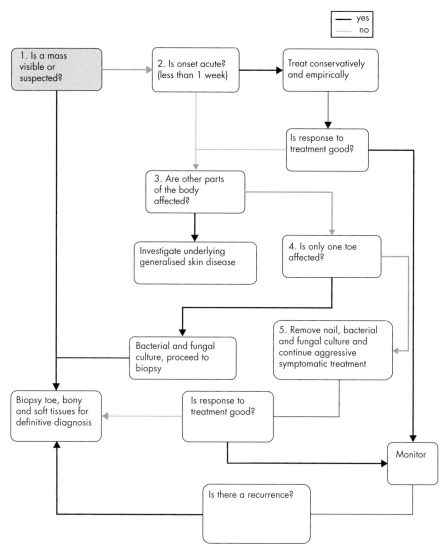

Figure 18.1 Management of nail and claw disease.

5 Where several toes are affected neoplasia is less likely
- Squamous cell carcinoma may affect multiple toes
- Neoplasia cannot be ruled out
- Paraneoplastic syndromes may affect multiple toes

Take skin scrapes for *Demodex* spp. bearing in mind that the mite can be hard to find on the feet. Biopsies should assist in diagnosis of this condition. Usually associated with more generalised pododermatitis.

Take samples for fungal culture. Dermatophytosis restricted to the toes is relatively common. Removed toe nails can be used for fungal culture.

Bacterial culture is less likely to be rewarding as the area is likely to be contaminated and intact pustules are rare.

Biopsy the toe. Either biopsy technique may be used although amputation is necessary if neoplasia is suspected.

18.1.1 TREATMENT OF COMMON CLAW AND NAIL DISEASES (SEE SECTION 5)

Although the treatment of these conditions is the same as for when other parts of the skin are affected, the special anatomy of these areas makes the treatment more challenging and the prognosis is more guarded. Aggressive appropriate treatment should always be maintained for some weeks beyond clinical cure on the first occasion of treatment to reduce the incidence of relapse.

Whilst topical treatments are always beneficial, they should be restricted to washes and rinses. The use of creams, ointments and salves should be avoided as the patient will lick them off, resulting in self-trauma.

Occlusal dressings are infrequently indicated.

Topical treatments will increase patient comfort considerably as well as reducing the duration of systemic treatments significantly.

Bacterial paronychia
- Can be transient and mild especially following trauma requiring only topical treatments with washes
- Persistent and recurrent cases benefit from removal of the nail
- Long courses of systemic antibiotics may be required
- Bacterial infection may be secondary to other underlying factors, so thorough investigation of persistent and recurrent cases is essential

Immune-mediated disease
Pemphigus foliaceus (Figures 18.2 and 18.3)
- May affect only the feet or include other parts of skin
- May be challenging to diagnose on biopsy
- Topical treatments and washes are beneficial in removing excess scale
- Address secondary pyoderma

Lupoid onychodystrophy (Figure 18.4)
- May be a transient mild disorder
- Do no harm with treatment
- Vitamin E has been used in mild cases. This may be combined with zinc and essential fatty acid supplementation
- Nicotinamide/tetracycline combinations have been used with some success
- Glucocorticoids effective in more severe cases, but have side-effects and are contraindicated in dermatophytosis and demodicosis, so should only be used when a definitive diagnosis has been made
- Azathioprine use should be restricted to the most severe cases that do not respond to other safer treatments

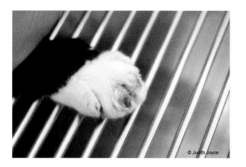

Figure 18.2 Nail bed lesions in pemphigus foliaceus in a cat.

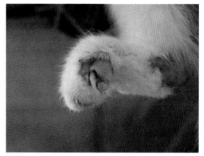

Figure 18.3 Nail bed lesions in a cat with drug eruption resembling pemphigus foliaceus.

Dermatophytosis
- Prognosis more guarded where the nails are involved
- Use of washes and rinses mandatory (enilconazole is toxic to cats)

Demodicosis
- Biopsy may be necessary for diagnosis
- Amitraz treatment of choice; however, some cases remain refractory to treatment or are recurrent
- Oral ivermectin regimes and milbemycin have been used off label with some success in non-responsive or recurrent cases
- Systemic antibacterials essential until beyond clinical cure
- Some refractory cases may respond to off label use of other drugs
- May occur as a complication of atopic dermatitis in patients on long-term anti-inflammatory treatments

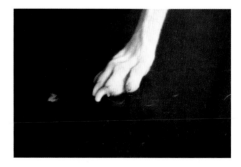

Figure 18.4 Nail loss and distortion caused by lupoid onychodystrophy.

18.2 MANAGEMENT OF FOOTPAD DISEASE

Figure 18.5 outlines the management of footpad lesions. The numbers in the text refer to the numbers on the figure.

1 Footpad lesions in the absence of other signs are relatively uncommon.

The Foot

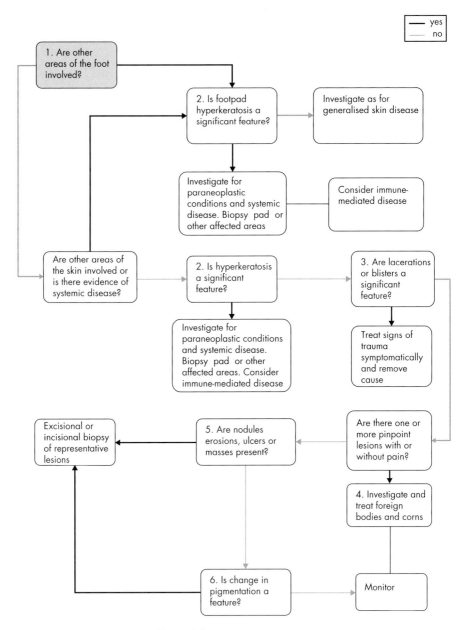

Figure 18.5 Management of footpad disease.

2 Footpad hyperkeratosis is a common finding, often as part of a generalised skin
   condition such as pemphigus foliaceus (Figure 18.6) or in systemic disease, such
   as superficial necrolytic dermatitis (hepatocutaneous syndrome, metabolic epidermal
   necrosis, necrolytic migratory erythema). Although footpad hyperkeratosis can
   occur as a localised disease, or in combination with nasal keratosis, it should be
   regarded as a warning sign of more significant disease.

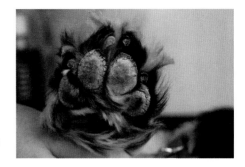

Figure 18.6 Footpad hyperkeratosis in a spaniel with pemphigus foliaceus.

3 Footpad trauma is perhaps the most common cause of footpad lesions. It can occur as a result of sharp trauma where lacerations occur. Blisters and erosions are frequently found in dogs who accompany their owners while jogging on hard surfaces or who obsessively play tug-of-war. Hot tarmac can also cause blisters.

4 Footpad foreign bodies are very common and easily missed. The entry wound may be very small and the foreign body not visible to the naked eye. Glass and other sharp hard objects are usually the cause. Corns, foreign body reactions to keratin, present similarly although there is often a longer duration of signs. In both cases there is usually well localised discomfort and the patient often presents with lameness. The treatment is general anaesthetic and surgical excision/removal.

Corns are relatively common on the third and fourth (weight bearing digits) of active sighthounds. The treatment of choice is surgical removal, but recurrence is common.

5 Nodules and masses are indicative of neoplasia, hyperplasia and in the cat, plasma cell pododermatitis (Figures 18.7 and 18.8). Masses may often be flattened or ulcerated on the footpad and therefore less identifiable. It is important that any lesion that any suspected mass or nodule is biopsied early.

6 Changes in pigmentation should be investigated early. They may be associated with neoplasia or immune-mediated conditions although they are also commonly associated with trauma and scarring.

Principles of treatment of footpad lesions

- If it is possible to take samples representative of the disease from areas other than the footpad, do so

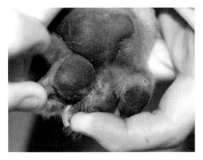

Figure 18.7 Swelling of multiple digital and metacarpal footpads in a Greyhound.

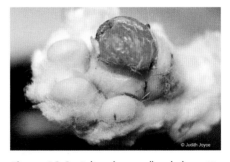

Figure 18.8 Feline plasma cell pododermatitis.

The Foot

- Footpad wounds bleed profusely and can be slow to heal
- It is easy to miss representative lesions when taking biopsies
- Histopathological interpretation of footpad skin is challenging
- Foreign bodies and corns should be ruled out as a cause at an early stage, especially in patients who present with lameness and racing or active sighthounds
- Consider analgesia. Weight bearing lesions may be painful
- Aggressive medical treatment is frequently required
- Topical treatments will always be a beneficial adjunct, also useful palliatively
- Foot coverings will help to protect the foot and increase contact time of topical treatments
- Review diagnosis in cases of poor response

18.3   PODODERMATITIS

Occurs in two main forms:
- Generalised erythema
- Interdigital fistulae

1 Generalised pedal erythema, caused by:

1   Ectoparasites (Figure 18.9)
2   Hypersensitivity dermatitis (Figures 18.10 and 18.11)
3   Immune-mediated disease (Figure 18.12)
4   Contact irritant reaction, e.g. road salt
5   Stuck on annoying substance, e.g. chewing gum
6   Minor trauma
7   Existence of psychogenic problems is controversial, e.g. habit and displacement activity

2 Interdigital fistulae ('interdigital cysts'), caused by:

1   Progression of generalised pedal erythema
2   Foreign body
3   Demodicosis
4   Dermatophytosis
5   Endocrine disease
6   Breed predisposition, e.g. English Bull Terrier and German Shepherd Dog

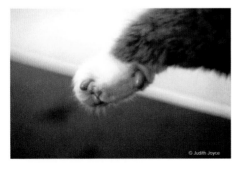

Figure 18.9   Ticks attached to cat's foot.

The Foot

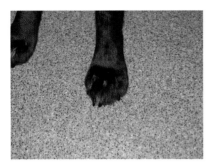

Figure 18.10 Pododermatitis in a Labrador Retriever with atopic dermatitis.

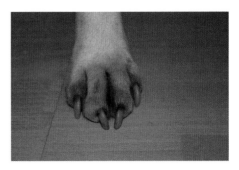

Figure 18.11 Saliva staining and *Malassezia* dermatitis in a Labrador Retriever with atopic dermatitis.

18.3.1 MANAGEMENT OF PEDAL ERYTHEMA

The management of pedal erythema is outlined in Figure 18.13. The numbers on the figure refer to the numbers in the text.

1 Pedal erythema occurs most commonly as either an acute local irritation or as part of a generalised skin disease. Some cases of hypersensitivity dermatitis may present with only signs of pododermatitis. Chronic or recurrent cases of pododermatitis should be thoroughly investigated and the underlying cause addressed if a single course of appropriate symptomatic treatment is not curative.

2 It is important that causes such as foreign body reaction or the presence of deep pyoderma/furunculosis are identified at an early stage. Examination under general anaesthesia and biopsy are advisable at an early stage if these conditions cannot be ruled out in the consulting room. It is also important that cases of pedal erythema are treated appropriately so that they do not progress to interdigital fistulae.

3 Generalised foot chewing, especially of one foot, may occur in the presence of a primary lesion. The foot should be examined carefully for the presence of hairballs or sticky items such as chewing gum on first presentation. Any nodule or ulcer should be biopsied at an early stage.

The Foot

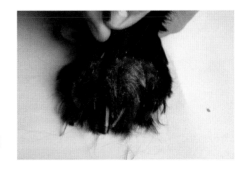

Figure 18.12 Pododermatitis in a spaniel with pemphigus foliaceus.

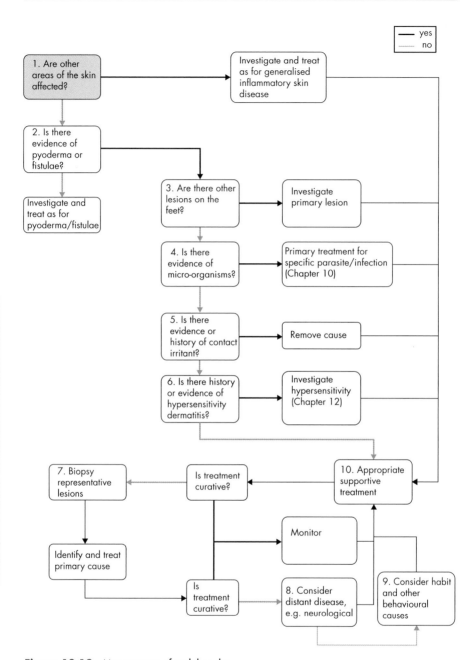

Figure 18.13 Management of pedal erythema.

4   The foot is a predilection site for many micro-organisms
   • History and clinical examination should reveal the presence of *Neotrombicula* reaction
   • History and clinical examination should reveal *Pelodera* and hookworm
   • Skin scrapes for *Sarcoptes* spp. and *Demodex* spp.
   • Fungal examination and culture for dermatophytosis

- Biopsy may be necessary for other micro-organisms
- Bacterial infection is likely to be secondary
- *Malassezia* dermatitis

5 Contact irritant reaction is common in foot disease. A careful history and clinical examination should reveal the likelihood of contact irritant reaction. Road grit and salt may be quite irritant to some dogs in winter and accumulations of snow and ice may cause persistent foot licking even after they have melted.

6 Hypersensitivity dermatitis is frequently associated with foot licking and chewing. The only presenting sign may be foot chewing in some cases.

7 In chronic or recurrent cases a biopsy should be performed to identify the primary cause and the initial diagnosis should be reviewed.

8 Some internal diseases can cause foot chewing, for example referred sensations in neurological disease or lethal acrodermatitis, acral mutilation syndrome.

9 Behavioural causes should only be considered when physical causes have been eliminated. Proposed mechanisms:
- Habituation – foot chewing remains a habit after removal of the initiating cause
- Dissociative behaviour – foot chewing occurs in the presence of another noxious stimulus
- Obsessive/compulsive behaviour

10 Appropriate supportive treatment is always beneficial.
1 Identify the underlying cause
2 Consider systemic antipruritic treatment – glucocorticoids can be used where not contraindicated
3 Foot rinsing and drying after walks removes contact irritants
4 Adjunctive topical washes and rinses to remove micro-organisms
5 Aggressive topical and systemic antibacterial treatments where indicated
6 Hair clipping to reduce skin humidity and increase contact of topical treatments
7 Occlusal dressings and boots to reduce self-trauma

18.3.2 MANAGEMENT OF INTERDIGITAL FISTULAE

Figure 18.14 outlines the management of interdigital fistulae and deep pyoderma. The numbers on the figure refer to the numbers in the text.

1 Other areas of the skin are often affected, for example, in pyoderma secondary to hypersensitivity dermatitis and German Shepherd Dog deep pyoderma/furunculosis. As the interdigital areas of the feet are the most resistant to treatment, lesions may persist here when those in other areas have resolved. Where only the feet are affected, especially if only one foot is affected interdigital foreign bodies must be ruled out at an early stage.

2 Draining tracks. In the presence of draining tracks or bullae foreign bodies must be ruled out first. The presence of more than one lesion does not rule out the possibility of foreign body reaction. A thorough examination of draining tracks can only be carried out under general anaesthetic.

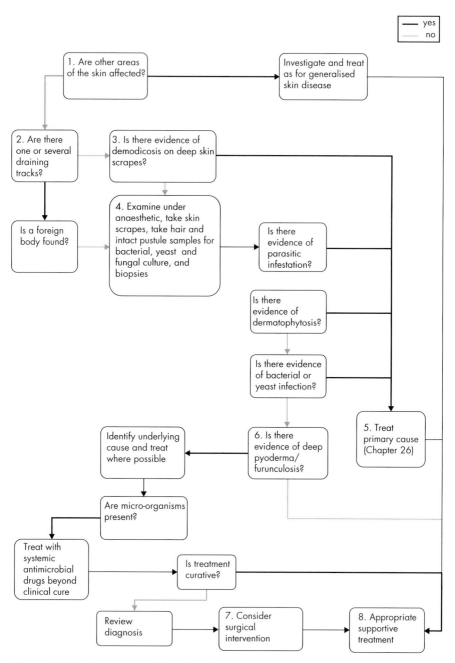

Figure 18.14 Management of interdigital fistulae.

The Foot

3   Pododemodicosis may be difficult to diagnose. Several deep skin scrapings should
     be taken before examination under anaesthetic as severe pododemodicosis may
     result in deep pyoderma/furunculosis and draining tracks. A negative skin scrape
     does not rule out a diagnosis of demodicosis as mites are often difficult to find on
     skin scrapings from the feet.

4   Further investigation for micro-organisms. If mites are not found, thorough
     examination of the lesions under general anaesthetic is mandatory. Samples for
     fungal, bacterial and yeast examination and culture can be taken and biopsy
     samples should be taken. Biopsy will reveal the presence of *Demodex* mites.

5   The primary cause should be addressed where possible. Any micro-organisms found
     should be treated appropriately until beyond clinical cure (see Chapter 26). Foot
     lesions generally require longer courses of treatment than other areas and there is
     more likely to be a recurrence of signs. Adequate supportive treatment is essential
     beyond clinical cure.

6   Deep pyoderma/furunculosis. If evidence of deep pyoderma/furunculosis is found
     the prognosis for cure is guarded to poor. Efforts to identify and treat the underly-
     ing cause should be renewed. In breeds who are predisposed to the condition (espe-
     cially English Bull Terrier and German Shepherd Dog pyoderma, long-term control
     measures are generally needed, including long-term systemic antibacterial courses
     in many cases).

7   Surgery should be considered in poorly responsive cases. In non-responsive or
     recurrent cases surgical podoplasty can be performed. This is only likely to be cura-
     tive where lesions are restricted to the interdigital areas, although it may aid in the
     control of other cases. It is, however, a demanding surgical technique and the advice
     of a surgeon should be sought.

8   Adequate supportive treatment
     • Systemic antibiotic therapy, based on the results of bacterial culture and sensi-
       tivity tests
     • Adjunctive topical treatments with antibacterial washes and shampoos
     • Regular rinsing of feet to increase comfort
     • Occlusal dressings and boots to reduce self-trauma should be used with caution
     • Consider analgesia, especially in cases of lameness
     • Regular review of diagnosis
     • If bacterial culture is negative, long-term suppression of furunculosis may be
       considered. Anti-inflammatory doses of glucocorticoids, or cyclosporin, may
       be effective, but great care is needed in their use (see Chapter 28).

Permanent scarring of the tissues increases the likelihood of recurrence and poor
response to treatment, so aggressive long-term control is usually necessary.

The Foot

Chapter 19

Skin Disease Affecting the Perianal Region

Perianal lesions appear very similar regardless of the underlying cause (see Figures 19.2 and 19.3).

19.1 MANAGEMENT OF PERIANAL SKIN DISEASE

Figure 19.1 outlines the management of perianal skin disease. The numbers in the text refer to the numbers on the figure.

Table 19.1 lists the causes of generalised skin disease where perianal skin is commonly affected.

Table 19.2 lists the causes of skin disease localised to the perianal skin.

1 Skin disease affecting other areas of the skin should be investigated as in Sections 2 and 3.

2 Anal sac disease
- Very common
- May be impacted, infected, abscessated or neoplastic

Clinical signs:
Most commonly perianal rubbing, licking or sudden jumping movement
Bleeding is often seen with abscessation and neoplasia
On presentation with perianal irritation, both anal sacs should be evacuated

- The contents should be examined
  - Impaction, clear liquid or grey/brown inspissated contents
  - Infection, purulent or sanguinous contents
  - Abscessation, pus and or blood with swelling inflammation and pain, possibly draining tracks
- The walls of the anal sacs examined carefully by palpation for thickening, especially irregular thickening and nodules
  - Regular thickening may be due to infection abscessation or early tumour formation
  - Irregular thickening may be due to chronic/recurrent infection, abscessation or tumour formation
  - Nodular thickening may be due to tumour or scar formation, investigation, staging, early removal and histopathological examination are indicated

If there are palpable thickenings of the anal sac wall or blood is evacuated removal of the gland should be considered.

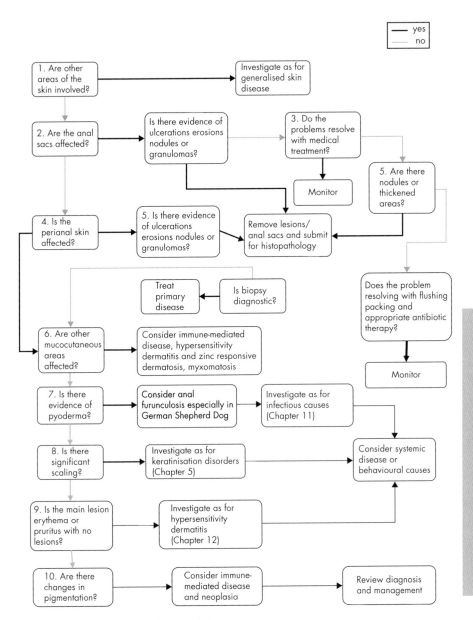

Figure 19.1 Management of perianal disease.

3 Recurrence of anal sac problems

If there is a good response to single treatment or the patient is presented on a regular basis for anal sac evaluation the condition should be monitored. If response is not complete, the anal sacs should be thoroughly examined under general anaesthesia.

a. The contents should be examined grossly as before
b. Bacterial and fungal culture should be considered

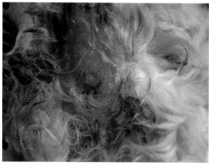

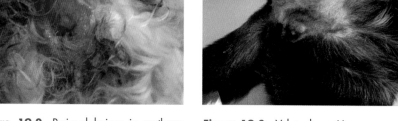

Figure 19.2 Perianal lesions in erythema multiforme in a Cocker Spaniel.

Figure 19.3 Vulvar dermatitis.

c. Anal sac walls should be palpated carefully
d. Removal of the anal sacs and histopathology should be considered
e. Thorough flushing of the sacs should be done after samples are taken
f. Antibiotic solutions are often instilled locally in addition to systemic treatment. This is an off label use of antibiotic but frequently successful

Table 19.1 Generalised skin disease in which perianal lesions commonly occur

Parasitic	Pelodera dermatitis
	Myiasis
Infection	FeLV dermatitis
	Myxomatosis
Hypersensitivity	Atopic dermatitis
	Contact irritant reaction
	Cutaneous adverse reaction to food
	'Hormonal hypersensitivity'
Keratinisation defects	Primary and secondary keratinisation defects
Pigmentary changes	Vitiligo
Endocrine	Adrenal hyperplasia like syndrome
Nodular and granulomatous diseases	Deep pyoderma/furunculosis
Immune mediated	Mucocutaneous pyoderma
	Pemphigus complex
	Bullous pemphigoid
	SLE
	Canine uveodermatologic syndrome
Neoplasia	Epitheliotrophic lymphoma
Paraneoplastic syndromes	Paraneoplastic pemphigus
	Hyperoestrogenism in testicular neoplasia
	Necrolytic migratory erythema
Nutritional	Zinc responsive dermatosis

Table 19.2 Skin diseases which are localised to the perianal region

Parasitic	No common examples
Infection	Tailfold intertrigo
Hypersensitivity	Contact irritant reaction
	? Cutaneous adverse reaction to food
Keratinisation defects	No common examples
Pigmentary changes	No common examples
Endocrine	No common examples
Nodular and granulomatous diseases	Neoplasia (see below)
	Perianal gland hyperplasia
	Anal furunculosis
Immune mediated	No common examples
Neoplasia	Perianal adenoma
	Anal gland carcinoma
	Other
Paraneoplastic syndromes	No common examples
Nutritional	Adverse cutaneous reaction to food?
Miscellaneous	Anal sac disease
	Anal furunculosis
	Anal licking (poodle)

Anal sac carcinoma
- May metastasise before clinically evident
- Hypercalcaemia often present
- Prognosis guarded

4 Diseases localised to the perianal skin
This is much more commonly associated with generalised skin disease with several important exceptions. Perianal lesions are often pronounced in myxomatosis and syphilis in the rabbit.

5 Nodular diseases of the perianal skin

Perianal adenoma
- Common
- More common in males, though do occur in females
- More common in older dogs
- Testosterone appears to be important in aetiology
- Many regress following castration

Perianal gland hyperplasia
- Common
- Similar clinical history
- Similar histopathology to perianal adenoma

Perianal gland adenocarcinoma
- Rare
- No response to castration
- More common in females
- More common in older male dogs
- Also – perianal gland epithelioma – rare

6 Perianal skin disease as part of a mucuocutaneous disease
- Perianal skin is frequently affected in generalised immune-mediated disease (see Figure 19.2)
- Hypersensitivity dermatitis may often affect some mucocutaneous areas (Figure 19.4)
- Mucocutaneous pyoderma
- Zinc responsive dermatosis

7 Evidence of pyoderma
- Pyoderma secondary to immune-mediated and hypersensitivity dermatitis
- Mucocutaneous pyoderma
- Tail fold intertrigo is a common secondary infection due to rubbing of skin folds in breeds of dog with tightly curled tails (Figure 19.5)
- Perivulvar dermatitis occurs with urine scalding in dogs where the folding of skin is excessive (e.g. obesity) or in dogs where the external genitalia is inadequately developed (Figure 19.3)

Skin Disease Affecting the Perianal Region

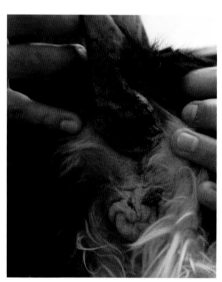

Figure 19.4 Perianal lesions in hypersensitivity dermatitis in a Cavalier Spaniel.

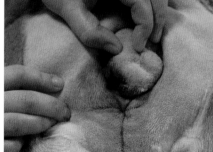

Figure 19.5 Corkscrew tail resulting in intertriginous dermatitis.

Anal furunculosis (Figure 19.6)
- Most common and refractory to treatment in German Shepherd Dog
- Prognosis guarded
- Aetiopathogenesis not fully understood
- May or may not be related to anal sac disease

Treatment
- Surgery – removal of all affected tissue with anal sacs
  - Cold steel
  - Cryosurgery
  - Laser surgery
- Medical – cyclosporin has proved effective in many cases (off label use), but long-term treatment is usually necessary to control the condition
  - May be combined with ketoconazole to reduce the cost of cyclosporin (off label use)
  - Fruit juices have been used to increase availability of cyclosporin and so reduce doses, but palatability issues as large volumes required, so generally impractical

See Chapters 26, 27.

8 Scaling
The perianal area is a commonly affected site in many scaling disorders, for example,
- Primary and secondary keratinisation defects
- Paraneoplastic syndromes
- Pemphigus complex
- Zinc responsive dermatosis
- Hypersensitivity dermatitis

It is unusual to find perianal scaling in isolation.

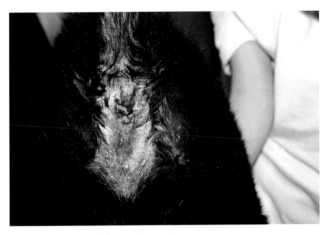

Figure 19.6 Anal furunculosis in German Shepherd Dog.

9 Hypersensitivity dermatitis

- The perianal area is a commonly affected site in hypersensitivity dermatitis, though rarely in isolation
- It has been suggested that this may be a predilected site in cutaneous adverse reaction to food
- It is a common site for contact irritant reaction

10 Changes in pigmentation

Changes in pigmentation are often undetected as the perianal area is not often inspected by the owner. Changes in pigmentation may be localised, for example, in vitiligo, or as part of a more generalised disease. Changes in pigmentation may also be a first presenting sign in neoplasia, so lesions should be biopsied at an early stage.

Skin Disease Affecting the
Perianal Region

Chapter 20

Ear Disease

The ear can be divided into the pinna, external ear canal, middle ear and inner ear.

This chapter will deal with diseases of the pinna and external ear canal. Surgical texts should be consulted for the management of middle and inner ear disease.

The pinna and external ear canal are lined with skin, so the general principles of the management of skin disease are the same.

The ear canal is a very specific environment, with the skin rolled into a cone. As aeration and access to this skin is restricted, the effects of inflammation, inflammatory products, scaling, greasiness and excess wax production are greatly magnified. The management of ear disease is therefore more challenging than many other less specialised areas of the skin.

20.1 MANAGEMENT OF PINNAL DISEASE

Table 20.1 lists skin diseases which commonly affect the pinna.

Table 20.1 Generalised skin diseases which commonly affect the pinna

Parasitic	*Otodectes* hypersensitivity dermatitis
	Demodicosis
	Sarcoptic mange
	Psoroptes cuniculi otitis in rabbits
	Lice, especially in dogs with pendulous ears
	Trombiculosis
	Spinous ear ticks
	Fly bites
	Flea bites, especially rabbit flea
Infection	Dermatophytosis
	Malassezia dermatitis
	Viral warts
	Pox virus
	Malassezia dermatitis
	Secondary pyoderma
	Various viral, protozoal, rickettsial diseases
Hypersensitivity	Atopic dermatitis
	Cutaneous adverse food reaction
	Parasitic hypersensitivity
Keratinisation defects	Primary and secondary keratinisation defects
	Sebaceous adenitis

(Continued)

Table 20.1 (Continued)

Pigmentary changes	Relatively rare but pinna can be affected
Endocrine	Hypothyroidism
	Hyperadrenocorticism
	Diabetes mellitus
Nodular and granulomatous diseases	Neoplasia
	Poxvirus
	Viral warts
	Idiopathic granuloma and pyogranuloma
Immune mediated	Pemphigus foliaceus
	Vasculitis
	Cold agglutinin disease
	Drug eruptions and reactions especially topical
	Bullous pemphigoid
	SLE
	Erythema multiforme
Neoplasia	Squamous cell carcinoma
	Mast cell tumour
	Histiocytoma
	Other
Paraneoplastic syndromes	Paraneoplastic pemphigus
	Paraneoplastic alopecia
	Necrolytic migratory erythema
Nutritional	Zinc responsive dermatosis
Miscellaneous	Psoriasiform lichenoid dermatosis in English Springer Spaniel
	Epidermolysis bullosa
	Familial canine dermatomyositis
	Hereditary lupoid dermatosis
	Lethal acral dermatitis
	Feline eosinophilic syndrome

Table 20.2 lists the causes of ear disease localised to the pinna.

Figure 20.1 outlines the management of pinnal disease. The numbers in the text refer to the numbers on the figure.

1 Generalised skin disease

If the pinnal lesions are part of a generalised skin disease this should be investigated.

Pruritus – see Chapter 4

Scaling – see Chapter 5

Hairloss – see Chapter 6 (Figure 20.2)

Pyoderma – see Chapter 7

Changes in pigmentation – see Chapter 8

Nodular disease – see Chapter 9

Ear Disease

Table 20.2 Conditions are localised to the pinna

Parasitic	Rabbit flea bite dermatitis
	Stick tight poultry flea
Infection	Dermatophytosis
	Viral warts
	Pox virus
Hypersensitivity	Atopic dermatitis
	Adverse cutaneous reaction to food
Keratinisation defects	Lichenoid keratosis
Pigmentary changes	Melanoderma and alopecia of Yorkshire Terriers
Nodular and granulomatous diseases	Pox virus
Immune mediated	? Pemphigus foliaceus
Neoplasia	Squamous cell carcinoma
	Plasmacytoma
	Mast Cell tumour
	Histiocytoma
Miscellaneous	Frost bite
	Actinic dermatitis
	Auricular chondritis
	Aural haematoma
	Idiopathic pinnal alopecia
	Preauricular feline alopecia
	Feline pinnal alopecia
	Familial vasculopathy
	Urticaria pigmentosa
	Arteriovenous fistula
	Iatrogenic pinnal folding in cats (glucocorticoids)

2 Concurrent otitis externa
- If there is also otitis externa present the condition should be investigated as for otitis externa

3 Ectoparasites (Figure 20.3)
- Ectoparasites are a common cause of pinnal disease
- Otocariasis and demodicosis may result in hairloss and excoriation due to self-trauma. More severe disease with severe crusting of the entire inner pinna may occur in rabbits (Figure 20.4)
- Scabies commonly affects the pinna as part of a more generalised disease
- Lice are commonly found on the pinna in louse infestation

4 Raised and ulcerative lesions
- Aural haematomas are readily identified by the presence of a soft to firm fluctuant swelling affecting all or part of the pinna. The aetiopathogenesis of this condition is clear and surgical drainage is usually required
- Masses and bleeding lesions should be biopsied at an early stage. Biopsy of the lesion demands careful surgery to prevent excessive bleeding and facilitate wound healing. Diathermy is useful

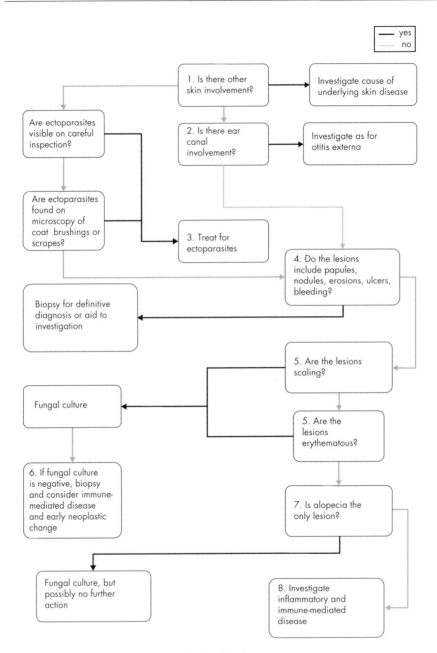

Figure 20.1 Management of diseases localised to the pinna.

5 Dermatophytosis

Fungal cultures should be taken from scaling lesions on the pinna, especially in cats as this is a predilection site for dermatophytosis.

6 Immune-mediated disease (Figures 20.5 and 20.6)

Where fungal cultures are negative immune-mediated disease and neoplasia should be considered. Early biopsy is mandatory to detect or rule out precancerous and malignant

Ear Disease

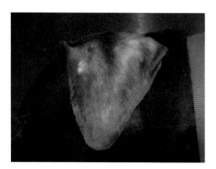

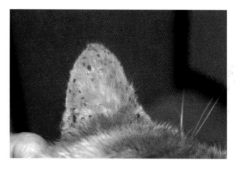

Figure 20.2 Pinnal hairloss associated with long-term glucocorticoid use.

Figure 20.3 Miliary lesions on cat pinna due to rabbit flea bite dermatitis.

change, indicative of early squamous cell carcinoma. Biopsy may also be useful in the diagnosis of immune-mediated disease. Although unusual to find only pinnal lesions in immune-mediated disease there is frequently minimal inflammation. Histopathology is not always diagnostic for immune-mediated disease.

7 Pattern alopecias
Several pattern alopecias affect the pinna. These are seen frequently in Dachshunds and Yorkshire Terriers and are benign. They do not respond to treatment. It is important to differentiate these from dermatophytosis.

8 Hypersensitivity dermatitis and other inflammatory diseases
Pinnal inflammation is one of the most common presenting signs of hypersensitivity dermatitis and pinnal lesions may occur in the absence of any other signs. Contact dermatitis due to topical applications should be considered in severe acute pinnal inflammation (see Chapter 4).

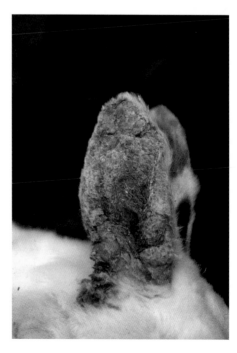

Figure 20.4 Severe scaling otitis due to *Psoroptes cuniculi* infestation in a rabbit.

Ear Disease

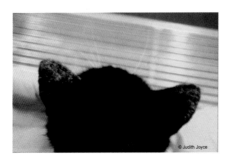

Figure 20.5 Pinnal lesions in feline pemphigus foliaceus.

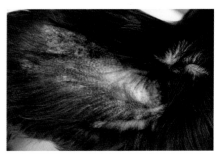

Figure 20.6 Pinnal lesions in pemphigus foliaceus in Cocker Spaniel.

20.2 MANAGEMENT OF ACUTE OTITIS EXTERNA (Figure 20.7)

1 Treat acute onset bacterial infections aggressively and promptly
2 Topical bacterial/steroid combinations appropriate
3 Identify triggering cause and remove (see Table 20.3) factors predisposing to otitis externa
4 General anaesthetic and ear flushing may be necessary
5 Investigate as chronic/recurrent otitis if appropriate therapy not curative

Prompt, aggressive, appropriate management of acute otitis externa will prevent progression to chronic recurrent otitis externa in many cases.

20.3 MANAGEMENT OF CHRONIC OR RECURRENT OTITIS EXTERNA (Figures 20.8 and 20.9)

There are three main principles underpinning the investigation of ear disease:
1 In all cases of chronic or persistent otitis externa the underlying cause should be identified and treated.
2 Otitis externa due to bacterial or yeast infection does not persist in healthy ears.
3 Surgery should be considered where the underlying cause cannot be treated effectively or where secondary changes cannot be reversed completely.

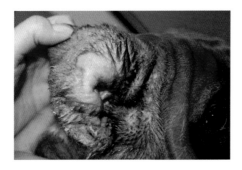

Figure 20.7 Acute moist dermatitis of pinna and external ear canal.

Ear Disease

Table 20.3 Factors predisposing to otitis externa

Anatomy	Narrow and tortuous external ear canal
	Excess hair or wax production
	Pendulous pinnae
Infection	Bacterial and yeast infections (usually secondary but significant)
	Internal disease predisposing to bacterial infection, for example, diabetes mellitus and HAC
Hypersensitivity dermatitis	Atopic dermatitis
	Cutaneous adverse reaction to food
	Parasitic hypersensitivity
Mechanical causes	Foreign body
	Water gaining access to the ear canal
	Administration of irritant or obstructive topical products
Ectoparasites	Otocariasis
	Tick
	Demodicosis
Environmental	Increased temperature and humidity resulting in bacterial or yeast infections
Neoplastic	Inflammatory polyp
	Carcinoma
Miscellaneous	Ceruminal gland hyperplasia

Steps in the investigation of otitis externa
Figure 20.10 outlines the steps in the investigation of chronic or recurrent otitis externa.

Investigation of underlying causes mandatory for successful treatment
Repeated use of polypharmaceutical topical products will always result in a long-term worsening of the condition.

1 Take a history and perform a full clinical examination
Identify generalised skin disease. The external ear canal is lined by skin in a challenging environment and otitis externa may often precede or be the only presenting sign of a more generalised problem.

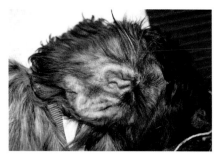

Figure 20.8 Changes in chronic otitis externa.

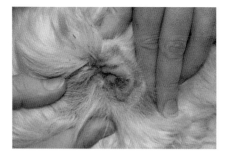

Figure 20.9 Changes to the ear canal in chronic otitis externa.

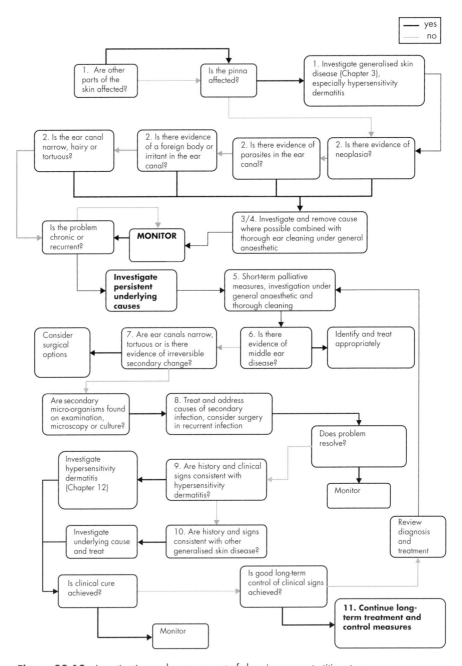

Figure 20.10 Investigation and management of chronic recurrent otitis externa.

Some systemic diseases may predispose to otitis externa, e.g. diabetes mellitus, and a number of diseases predispose to exfoliative dermatitis.

Information will also be gathered about the severity of the ear disease and the willingness of the client to investigate the underlying problem.

A thorough history will aid in the investigation of hypersensitivity dermatitis as an underlying cause.

2 A careful examination and evaluation of the ear canal in the consulting room

Where patient discomfort or lack of compliance precludes this the patient should be admitted for general anaesthesia and examination. Many causes of recurrent otitis persist due to inadequate examination of the ear canals. If general anaesthesia is necessary the full examination outlined below should be carried out.

The external ear canals should be examined under general anaesthetic

Sedation is rarely adequate in an inflamed ear canal and conscious examination in the consulting room is never adequate in more chronic cases.

Characterise the ear disease

State of the canal
- Narrow, tortuous
- Presence of hair and secretions
- Evidence of inflammation, ulceration
- Secondary change

Nature of exudate
- Ceruminous
- Dry, crumbly
- Dark, light
- Purulent
- Scale
- Presence of ear mites

Pinnal involvement, evidence of generalised skin disease

Take samples from ear canals

- Low power examination in liquid paraffin for ectoparasites, scale and debris
- High power examination of stained samples for rods, cocci and *Malassezia*
- Samples for microbiology. Use a proven laboratory for culture, identification and sensitivity testing. Don't wait for the results before starting treatment. Microbial infection is always secondary

Further investigations which may be considered while under general anaesthesia

- Consider investigation of presence of middle or inner ear disease
- Consider investigation of generalised skin disease
- Consider investigation of other internal disease

Consider treatment options while hospitalised

1 Remove and treat initiating causes
2 Thorough cleaning of the ear canal
3 Short-term palliative measures
4 Investigation and management of initiating disease
5 Long-term therapeutic options
6 Indications for surgery

3 Remove and treat the initiating cause where possible

Ear mites cannot always be identified macroscopically or even on examination of ear exudates microscopically, so where they cannot be excluded as a cause of otitis externa therapeutic trial using an ectoparasiticide should be considered.

Examine carefully for the presence of foreign bodies. Always check the other ear!

4 Thorough cleaning of the ear canal

- Hair, wax and exudate should be removed from the ear canals during the investigation
- Improve aeration of canals
- Remove irritant inflammatory products
- Improve contact of topical products

5 Short-term palliative measures

a. Inflamed ears will benefit from the short-term use of topical antibiotic and steroid combination treatments
b. Care should be exercised if the tympanic membrane may be ruptured
c. Consider patient comfort post-operatively
d. Short-term oral glucocorticoids may be beneficial
e. The use of ear wicks may be indicated (see Chapter 29.5)

6 Look for evidence of middle ear disease

It is important that the presence of middle ear disease is identified. Otitis externa will not respond to treatment in the presence of persisting middle ear disease.

Middle ear disease should be addressed at this stage.

7 Look for evidence of changes to the ear canal

If there is evidence of permanent secondary change or if the anatomy of the ear is such that the patient is likely to be predisposed to a recurrence of otitis externa, surgery should be considered.

8 Treat bacterial or yeast infection

Bacterial or yeast infections are nearly always secondary to changes in the external ear canal and its skin. However, once infection is established it can be self-perpetuating, so aggressive appropriate management of bacterial involvement is necessary (see Chapter 27.2).

If there is not a permanent response to a single course of appropriate antibacterial therapy based on culture and sensitivity results treatment should be reviewed.

Persisting underlying factors continue to predispose to infection and must be addressed.

The presence of *Pseudomonas* infection is strong evidence for a persisting underlying factor.

Persistent *Pseudomonas* infection causes significant damage to the ear canal which often necessitates surgery.

Consider MRSA, MRSI if not already identified.

Treat secondary infections aggressively using appropriate antimicrobials for long enough. Monitor progress with repeated cytological examinations (Chapter 27).

9 Hypersensitivity dermatitis

This is probably the most common cause of otitis externa in the dog and should be investigated as for generalised hypersensitivity dermatitis (see Chapter 12).

Hypersensitivity dermatitis should be suspected whenever there is pinnal involvement.

Hypersensitivity dermatitis most commonly presents as a generalised dermatitis, but in some cases only the ears may be affected or the ear pathology precedes other clinical signs.

Secondary complications may obscure the appearance of hypersensitivity dermatitis in chronic otitis externa.

The possibility of hypersensitivity dermatitis should be investigated and addressed at an early stage.

Long-term control of secondary complications, including surgery, may be required in many cases of otitis due to hypersensitivity dermatitis.

10 Investigate other skin and generalised diseases

Table 20.4 lists the generalised skin diseases which commonly predispose to otitis externa.

Other skin diseases, especially those which predispose to scaling, inflammation or secondary infections may cause otitis externa (see Chapters 4–9).

Other systemic disease, especially those which affect the immune system, or predispose to scaling inflammation or secondary infection may cause otitis externa.

This may be curative in many cases but due to the factors listed below long-term control measures are often required. This should include a regular review of persisting underlying causes and changes to the ear canal.

11 Long-term control of otitis externa

May be necessary because of:

1. Anatomical abnormalities or changes to the canal

- Anatomical limitations, such as long tortuous or narrow canals, pendulous pinnae or hairy ears
- Permanent secondary changes to the ear canal such as thickening and calcification of the canals and hyperplastic ceruminal glands
- Ceruminal gland hyperplasia
- Otitis results in hyperplasia and excess secretion
- Changed cerumen composition, watery and less flushing
- May take months to resolve after resolution of otitis

2. Owner compliance regarding investigation or treatment

- Owners may decline investigation of the underlying cause
- The secondary role of bacterial infection should be discussed before resorting to long-term medical management
- Regular ear cleaning is integral to the long-term management of chronic or recurrent otitis externa and some patients may become less compliant, especially where inflammation is poorly controlled and the procedure causes discomfort

3. Incomplete control of the underlying cause

- Hypersensitivity dermatitis
- Systemic disease
- Generalised skin disease

Table 20.4 Generalised skin and systemic diseases commonly predisposing to otitis externa

Generalised skin disease	Ectoparasites	Scabies
		Demodicosis
		Otocariasis
	Micro-organisms	Dermatophytosis
		Deep pyoderma
	Hypersensitivity dermatitis	Parasitic hypersensitivity
		Atopic dermatitis
		Adverse cutaneous reaction to food
		Other
	Immune mediated	Pemphigus foliaceus
		Drug eruption
		SLE
	Primary and secondary keratinisation defects	Primary genetic keratinisation defect
		Vitamin A responsive dermatosis
		Zinc responsive dermatosis
		Hypersensitivity dermatitis
		Paraneoplastic syndromes
	Primary and secondary skin neoplasia	Epitheliotrophic lymphoma
		Multiple primary masses
		Metastatic disease
		Paraneoplastic syndromes
Systemic disease	Endocrine disease	Diabetes mellitus
		Hyperadrenocorticism
		Hypothyroidism
	Immunosuppressive disease	Congenital or inherited disorders
		Lymphoproliferative disorders
		Viral infection
	Neoplasia	Paraneoplastic syndromes
		Secondary metastatic disease

4. Flares of the initiating disease
- Seasonal flare
- Secondary infection
- Environmental change

5. Environment of the ear canal
The cone shape of the ear canal results in accumulation of grease, wax, sweat, hair and inflammatory products that can more readily be removed from other areas of the skin.

Factors which must be constantly addressed and reviewed long term
1 Failure to identify and address the underlying cause of acute otitis externa
2 Failure to address anatomical factors favouring dark, damp environment in the ear and obstruction of the ear canal
3 Inflammation causing occlusion and thickening of the external ear canal

Ear Disease

4 Inflammation causing hyperplasia of the ceruminal glands, hence overproduction of cerumen
5 Altered composition of cerumen caused by overactivity of ceruminal glands
6 Accumulation of scale and ceruminal gland secretions
7 Inflammatory cytokines produced in inflammation causing increased erythema, inflammation and exudation
8 Ideal environment produced by 1–6 favour bacterial and yeast colonisation
9 Inflammatory cytokines produced in secondary bacterial and yeast infections

Regime for long-term control
Regular ear cleaning
1 Removes cerumen, exudate and debris from canal
2 Removes irritant inflammatory products
3 Improves contact of topical products
4 Antimicrobial action of low pH products
5 Astringent
6 Flushing effect with some ear cleaners
Regular assessment for flare factors
Regular review of underlying causes
Judicious use of oral glucocorticoids
1 Antipruritic effect in inflammatory ear disease
2 Treatment of ceruminal gland hyperplasia
3 Care in the presence of infection, systemic or generalised skin disease
Occasional use of topical antibiotic/glucocorticoids in the presence of flares
1 Short infrequent courses only
2 If a short course of any preparation does not work the case should be reviewed, alternatives should not be used

Use of ear wicks
Ear wicks have been used with some success in chronic recurrent otitis externa where secondary bacterial infection and inflammation are significant. The use of ear wicks is detailed in Chapter 29.

Surgery
1 Most effective when considered early in the ear disease before severe irreversible secondary change has taken place.
2 Surgery should always be considered where the underlying cause can be controlled but not cured and control is less than 100% effective.
3 Surgery should be considered as a useful adjunct in long-term therapeutic control measures.
4 Surgery may be curative in many cases where medical treatment would be ineffective.
• Anatomical defects
• Chronic or persistent infection
• Ceruminal hyperplasia
• Aural polyps or tumours
5 Surgery is frequently necessary when irreversible secondary change has taken place, despite the initiating cause being addressed. This is particularly the case where secondary infections have become well established.

Chapter 21
Periocular Skin Disease

Periocular lesions are often very similar whatever the underlying cause. See Figures 21.1 and 21.2.

Table 21.1 lists conditions where the periorbital skin is commonly affected.

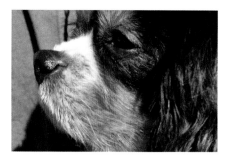

Figure 21.1 Periorbital and muzzle lesions in Cavalier Spaniel with atopic dermatitis.

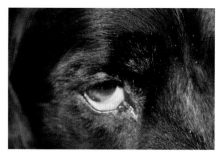

Figure 21.2 Periorbital lesions in English Springer Spaniel with pemphigus foliaceus.

Table 21.1 Conditions in which periocular lesions commonly occur

Parasitic	Scabies, demodicosis
Infection	FeLV dermatitis
	Myxomatosis
Hypersensitivity	Atopic dermatitis
	Cutaneous adverse food reaction
	Scabies hypersensitivity
Keratinisation defects	Primary and secondary keratinisation defects
Pigmentary changes	Vitiligo
	Lentigo simplex of ginger cats
Endocrine	
Nodular and granulomatous diseases	Idiopathic sterile granuloma and pyogranuloma
Immune-mediated	Pemphigus complex
	SLE
Neoplasia	Epitheliotrophic lymphoma
Paraneoplastic syndromes	Paraneoplastic pemphigus
	Necrotic migratory erythema
Nutritional	Biotin deficiency
	Zinc responsive dermatosis
Miscellaneous	Juvenile cellulitis
	Canine uveodermatologic syndrome
	Canine familial dermatomyositis

Table 21.2 Conditions localised to the periocular area

Parasitic	No common conditions
Infection	Sialodacryoadenitis virus in rats
Hypersensitivity	Occasionally atopic dermatitis
Keratinisation defects	No common conditions
Pigmentary changes	Lentigo simplex of ginger cats
	Familial leukotrichia of Siamese cats
Endocrine	No common conditions
Nodular and granulomatous diseases	See Neoplasia
Immune-mediated	No common conditions
Neoplasia	Squamous cell carcinoma
	Basal cell tumour
	Mast cell tumour
	Papillomas
	Meibomian gland tumours
	Melanoma
	Dermoid
	Histiocytoma
	Lymphoma
Paraneoplastic syndromes	No common conditions
Nutritional	No common conditions
Miscellaneous	Entropion
	Ectropion
	Trichiasis
	Distachiasis
	Hordoleum
	Chalazion
	Excess epiphora
	Prolapsed third eyelid gland `cherry eye´

Table 21.2 lists common skin conditions localised to the periorbital area.

21.1 MANAGEMENT OF PERIOCULAR DISEASE

Figure 21.3 outlines the management of periocular disease. The numbers in the text refer to the numbers on the figure.

Eye lesions or rubbing or discomfort can be caused by:
- Ocular disease
- Eyelid abnormalities
- Periocular skin disease
1 **Periocular lesions** are common in many generalised skin diseases (Figure 21.4). There are, however, some important abnormalities which affect the eyelids alone.

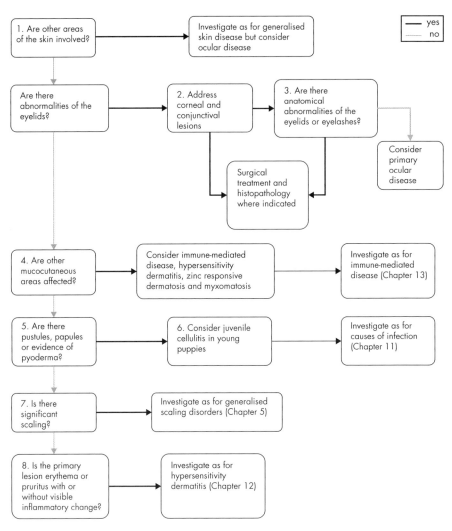

Figure 21.3 Management of periocular disease.

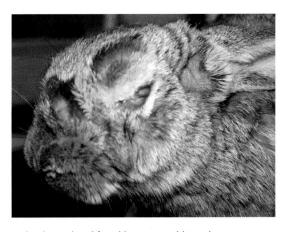

Figure 21.4 Periorbital, nasal and facial lesions in rabbit with myxomatosis.

2   **Ocular disease.** A full ocular examination should be carried out to investigate the possibility of primary or secondary ocular disease. Ocular lesions should be treated whether primary or secondary to prevent worsening and to improve patient comfort.

3   **Eyelid abnormalities** can be of several types and are commonly associated with periocular irritation.
    - Anatomical eyelid abnormalities, such as ectropion, entropion
    - Hair abnormalities such as ectopic cilia and distichiasis
    - Eyelid masses

    If these primary causes are not addressed it will be difficult to control periorbital disease.

    Eyelid masses should be approached in the same way as other neoplastic disease (see Chapter 16). However, wound closure after mass removal may be challenging and referral to a surgeon/ophthalmologist should be considered.

4   **Mucocutaneous lesions.** The skin around the eyes is commonly affected in skin conditions with a mucocutaneous distribution, for example
    - Immune-mediated disease (see Chapter 13)
    - Mucocutaneous pyoderma (see Chapters 11 and 13)
    - Zinc responsive dermatosis (see Chapter 17)
    - Paraneoplastic syndromes (see Chapter 16)
    - Myxomatosis in rabbits (see Chapter 11)

    Periocular lesions are very frequently seen in hypersensitivity dermatitis.

5   **Pustules and papules**
    - May indicate the presence of a primary infection
    - Commonly occur secondary to an inflammatory or immune-mediated condition (see Chapter 11)

6   **Juvenile cellulitis in puppies**
    - Uncertain aetiopathogenesis
    - Periocular and eyelid lesions occur as part of a syndrome including facial lesions, lymphadenopathy, pyrexia, depression in young puppies
    - Pustules often sterile
    - Responsive to glucocorticoids

7   **Scaling.** It is unusual to find periocular scaling in isolation. The periocular area is a commonly affected site in many scaling disorders such as:
    - Primary and secondary keratinisation defects (Chapter 5)
    - Paraneoplastic syndromes (Chapters 16, 17)
    - Pemphigus complex (Chapter 13)
    - Zinc responsive dermatosis (Chapter 17)
    - Hypersensitivity dermatitis (Chapter 12)

8   **Hypersensitivity dermatitis.** The periocular area is a commonly affected site in hypersensitivity dermatitis, though rarely in isolation.

    It has been suggested that this may be a predilected site in cutaneous adverse reaction to food but there is little firm evidence to support this.

    Common site for contact irritant reaction, including reactions to topical therapeutic agents.
    See Chapter 12.

Chapter 22

Dermatoses Affecting the Muzzle

The muzzle includes the haired skin of the face around the nose and muzzle, and the mucocutaneous structures of the lips and nasal planum.

22.1 MANAGEMENT OF THE HAIRED SKIN OF THE MUZZLE

Table 22.1 lists the common diseases affecting the haired skin of the muzzle.

Table 22.2 lists the common diseases localised to the muzzle.

Figure 22.1 outlines the management of the haired skin of the muzzle and lips. The numbers in the text refer to the numbers on the figure.

1   **Generalised skin disease.** The nose and mouth areas are commonly affected in generalised skin disease. A list of generalised dermatoses where lesions commonly occur around the nose and mouth is shown in Table 22.1.

2   **The nasal planum** is a very specialised area of skin which is frequently affected in mucocutaneous conditions (see Figure 22.2).

Table 22.1 Skin diseases in which muzzle lesions can occur

Parasitic	Demodicosis
Infection	Dermatophytosis
	Blastomycosis
	Cryptococcosis
	Aspergillosis
	FeLV dermatitis
	Distemper
	Canine papilloma virus
	Canine ehrlichiosis
	Leishmaniosis
	Myxomatosis
	Rabbit 'syphilis'
	Pox virus
Hypersensitivity	Atopic dermatitis
	Cutaneous adverse reaction to food
Keratinisation defects	Primary and secondary keratinisation defects
	Ichthyosis
	Follicular cornification disorder
Pigmentary changes	Vitiligo
	DLE
	Mucocutaneous hypopigmentation
Endocrine	

Nodular and granulomatous diseases	Idiopathic granuloma and pyogranuloma
Immune mediated	Pemphigus complex
	Epidermolysis bullosus acquisita
	SLE
	DLE
	Juvenile cellulitis
Neoplasia	Epitheliotrophic lymphoma
Paraneoplastic syndromes	Paraneoplastic pemphigus
	Necrolytic migratory erythema
Nutritional	Zinc responsive dermatosis
Miscellaneous	Mucocutaneous pyoderma
	Angio-oedema
	Vasculitis
	Cryoglobulinaemia
	Cryofibronogenaemia
	Familial canine dermatomyositis
	Lethal acrodermatitis of English Bull Terrier
	Snake bite

Table 22.2 Skin diseases which are localised to the muzzle

Parasitic	
Infection	Nasal furunculosis/deep pyoderma
	Dermatophytosis
Hypersensitivity	
Keratinisation defects	Nasal hyperkeratosis
	Feline acne
	Canine 'acne'
Pigmentary changes	DLE
	Melanoderma and alopecia of Yorkshire Terriers
	Lentigo simplex of ginger cats
Endocrine	
Nodular and granulomatous diseases	Idiopathic granuloma and pyogranuloma
Immune mediated	DLE
Neoplasia	Squamous cell carcinoma
	Plasmacytoma
	Melanoma
Paraneoplastic syndromes	
Nutritional	
Miscellaneous	Familial vasculopathy
	Canine nasal solar dermatitis
	Lip fold dermatitis
	Bold nose and sore nose in gerbil

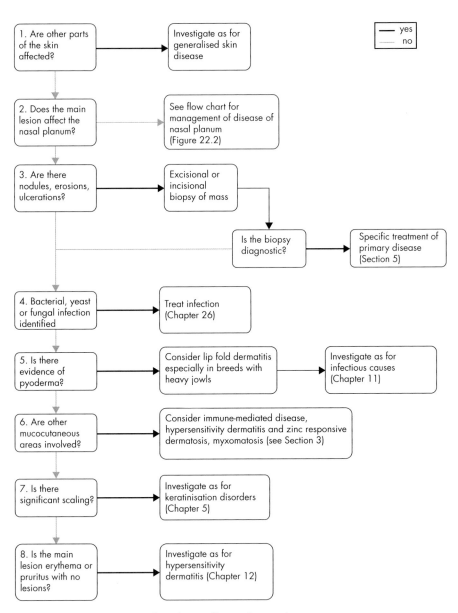

Figure 22.1 Management of conditions affecting the muzzle.

3   **Nodular or erosive lesions** should be biopsied at an early stage to diagnose or elimi-
    nate the possibility of neoplastic disease (Figure 22.3).

4   **Dermatophytosis.** The nose and mouth are predilection sites for dermatophytosis
    as this area is used to investigate (terriers in rabbit holes) and feed (pups feed-
    ing from mother). Fungal culture is mandatory in scaling and non-responsive
    lesions.

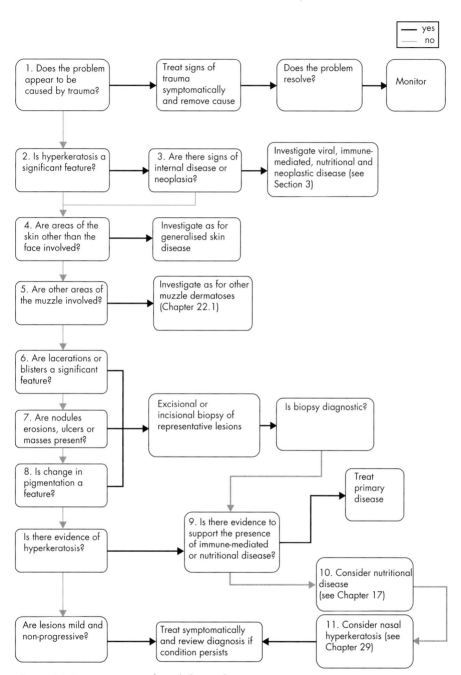

Figure 22.2 Management of nasal planum disease.

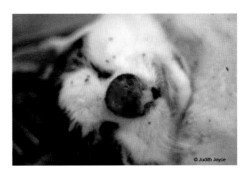

Figure 22.3 Squamous cell carcinoma in a cat.

5   Infection
- Nasal pyoderma/furunculosis (Figure 22.4)
  - ○ Acute onset infection of dorsal muzzle
  - ○ Trauma or sting may be involved in pathogenesis
  - ○ Rapid response to antibiotics (see Chapter 27.2)
  - ○ Analgesia is often required
- Lip fold dermatitis
  - ○ Heavy jowled breeds especially Cocker, Clumber, Sussex and Springer spaniels
  - ○ Often presented as halitosis (but usually more foul smelling)
  - ○ Mild to moderate cases respond to medical management (see Chapters 27.2, 29)
  - ○ Lip fold excision indicated in non-responsive, recurrent and severe cases

6   Nasal and lip lesions as part of a mucocutaneous disease
- Lesions can be scaling erythematous papular, pustular, erosive or loss of pigmentation
- Immune-mediated skin disease (see Chapter 13)
- Hypersensitivity dermatitis (see Chapter 12)
- Mucocutaneous pyoderma (see Chapter 11)
- Zinc responsive dermatosis (see Chapter 17)
- Myxomatosis (see Chapter 11)

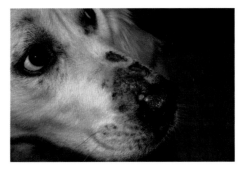

Figure 22.4 Nasal pyoderma/furunculosis.

7   Scaling disorders of the muzzle

- The muzzle is frequently affected both in generalised and localised diseases
- DLE
- Zinc responsive dermatosis
- Dermatophytosis
- Pemphigus diseases (Figure 22.5)
- Necrolytic migratory erythema
- Hypersensitivity dermatitis

8   Hypersensitivity dermatitis

- The muzzle is frequently affected in hypersensitivity dermatitis, usually as part of a more generalised skin disease

Feline acne

- Clinical lesions of comedones with variable inflammation and sometimes secondary infection on the chin
- May occur as part of many generalised inflammatory diseases or keratinisation defects
- Localised keratinisation defect
- Secondary infection addressed before long-term control measures initiated
- Topical antibacterial, glucocorticoid or 'follicle flushing' treatments beneficial
- Systemic treatment rarely justified, often only a cosmetic problem
- Severe cases may respond to:
  - Investigation of underlying causes
  - Systemic antibiotic treatment followed by
  - Glucocorticoids
  - Retinoids – care should be exercised before considering these drugs in a relatively benign disease

Canine acne

- Usually presents as part of a more generalised folliculitis secondarily infected with bacteria or yeasts
- Comedones less frequently a feature
- Pruritus and secondary inflammation frequently a feature
- Treatment as for feline 'acne' but systemic treatment more frequently necessary

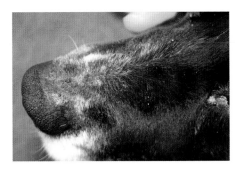

Figure 22.5   Nasal hairloss and scaling in pemphigus foliaceus.

Dermatoses Affecting the Muzzle

- Frequently part of a more generalised folliculitis
- Guarded prognosis for complete resolution in short term

(See Chapters 27.2, 29.)

Malassezia dermatitis

Usually a more generalised disease but may be localised to the muzzle and facial folds especially in short-nosed breeds of cat. (See Chapter 11.)

22.2 MANAGEMENT OF DISEASES AFFECTING THE NASAL PLANUM

The nasal planum is a highly specialised area of skin, characterised by a thickened epithelium, dense stratum corneum and rete ridges. For this reason histopathology should always be performed by an experienced veterinary dermatopathologist.

Figure 22.2 outlines the management of diseases of the nasal planum. The numbers in the text refer to the numbers on the figure.

1   Trauma
- The most common cause of conditions of the nasal planum is injury

2   Hyperkeratosis
- The second most common condition of the nasal planum is hyperkeratosis. Mild nasal hyperkeratosis can be treated symptomatically if:
  - Lesions are restricted to nasal planum
  - Lesions are mild and not resulting in clinical disease
  - It is non-progressive
  - A differential diagnosis and action plan has been discussed with owner

3   Internal disease
- Hyperkeratosis may be a sign of internal disease, although skin signs may occur before systemic signs become apparent. Common causes include:
  - Distemper
  - Nutritional dermatoses, e.g. zinc responsive dermatosis
  - Paraneoplastic syndromes
  - Immune-mediated disease

4   Generalised skin disease
- Nasal planum lesions frequently occur as part of a generalised skin disease

5   Facial skin disease
- Nasal planum lesions frequently occur as part of a facial skin disease

6   Trauma
- Lacerations of the nasal planum may occur as the result of injury, but these lesions should raise the suspicion of immune-mediated or neoplastic disease and should be biopsied if they do not respond to symptomatic treatment rapidly and permanently

7   Neoplasia
- Masses, erosions and ulcerations of the nasal planum should be biopsied at the earliest opportunity to investigate the possibility of neoplastic disease

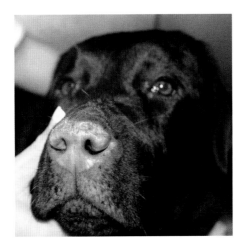

Figure 22.6 Crusting and loss of pigmentation in immune-mediated disease.

- Squamous cell carcinoma presenting as erythema or change in pigmentation followed by erosion is a common neoplasm of the nasal planum of the cat or dog (Figure 22.3)
- Other tumours are relatively uncommon

8 **Loss of pigmentation** of the nasal planum is the third most common presenting sign of nasal skin disease
- Secondary to trauma
- For unknown reasons in golden and Labrador Retrievers
- Associated with actinic dermatitis
- Associated with immune-mediated disease (Figure 22.6)
- An early sign of neoplasia

Early biopsy is essential in cases where trauma is not suspected as a cause to investigate the possibility of neoplastic disease.

9 **Immune-mediated lesions** of the nasal planum are relatively common
- DLE, exacerbated by sunlight
- Pemphigus complex

10 **The nasal planum may be affected in zinc responsive dermatosis**

11 **Nasal hyperkeratosis** is a common and benign thickening restricted to the nasal planum. This may lead to cracking and bleeding. There is no specific treatment; emollients and moisturisers may be effective (see Chapter 29).

Chapter 23

Management of Facial Lesions

Figure 23.1 outlines the management of facial lesions. The numbers in the text refer to the numbers on the figure.

1   Facial lesions are common in many generalised skin diseases Common problems are shown in bold in Table 23.1. These diseases are described in Sections 2 and 3. Common dermatoses which are localised to the face are listed in Table 23.2.

2   Lesions which affect the specialised areas of the face and head are covered in Chapters 21–23.

3   Nodular, raised or erosive lesions should be biopsied at an early stage, to rule out the possibility of neoplasia.
   Papilloma virus and feline pox virus lesions can be diagnosed on biopsy. Although rare conditions, these are frequently found on the head.
   Granulomatous lesions will also be differentiated from neoplasms on biopsy.

4   In cats the most common cause of erythematous raised lesions is eosinophilic plaque which has many causes, the most common of which is hypersensitivity dermatitis, including flea bite dermatitis (Chapter 4.4.2).

Where the appearance of the lesion is consistent with eosinophilic plaque, and there is no increased suspicion of neoplasia, short-term treatment for hypersensitivity dermatitis can be attempted.

Careful monitoring and frequent review is essential so that neoplasia is detected.

5   The face is a predilection site for cutaneous anaphylactic reaction, including reactions to bites and stings
   • Reactions can be localised or more generalised swellings, angioedoema, hives, or urticaria (Figures 2.30, 2.31)
   • Most patients respond very quickly to treatment with antihistamines (off label use) or glucocorticoids
   • Recurrent cases should undergo investigation for underlying causes
   • Patients with these lesions should be monitored carefully for signs of generalised anaphylactic reactions which may be life-threatening
   • Possibility of snake, fly and spider bites should also be considered, especially in terriers

6   The face is a common site for dermatophytosis, especially in terriers. Dermatophytosis should always be suspected in localised facial scaling.
   • *Malassezia* dermatitis frequently affects the face in cats

7   Pyoderma may occur secondary to many skin diseases, but facial lesions are usually only seen as part of a more generalised pattern. One exception is acute moist dermatitis which is frequently found on the cheek below the pinna in Labrador and golden retrievers and Rottweilers (Figure 23.2).

8   Intertrigo of the facial folds is a significant problem in short nosed breeds, especially when compounded by tear overflow.

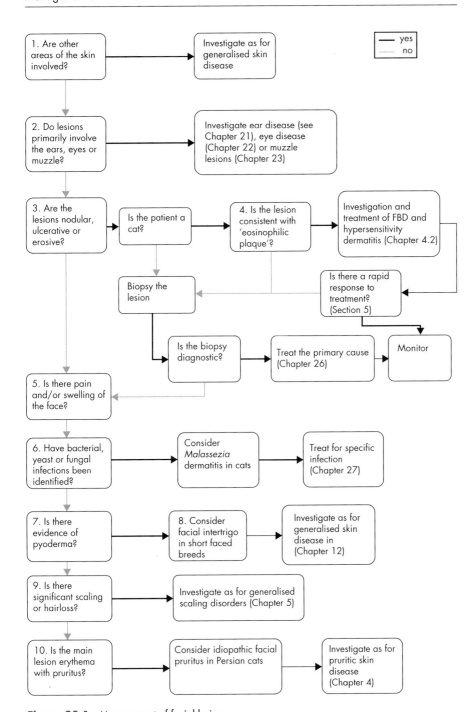

Figure 23.1 Management of facial lesions.

Table 23.1　Skin diseases which demonstrate facial lesions

Parasitic	**Otocariasis**
	Scabies
Infection	Feline TB
	Leprosy
	***Malassezia* dermatitis in cats**
	FeLV dermatitis
	FIV dermatitis
	Feline herpes virus
Hypersensitivity	**Atopic dermatitis**
	Parasitic hypersensitivity
	Adverse cutaneous reaction to food
Keratinisation defects	
Pigmentary changes	Vitiligo
Endocrine	
Nodular and granulomatous diseases	**Eosinophilic plaque**
Immune mediated	**Pemphigus complex**
	SLE
Neoplasia	Epitheliotrophic lymphoma
Paraneoplastic syndromes	Paraneoplastic pemphigus
	Necrolytic migratory erythema
Nutritional	**Zinc responsive dermatosis**
Miscellaneous	**Juvenile cellulitis**
	Insect and arachnid bites and stings
	Angio-oedema
	Cutaneous anaphylactic reaction
	Canine uveodermatologic syndrome
	Epidermolysis bullosa
	Familial canine dermatomyositis
	Hereditary lichenoid dermatosis
	Lethal acrodermatitis of EBT
	Feline hypereosinophilic syndrome

- Long-term topical maintenance treatment is indicated
- Surgery to remove the facial folds should be considered in non-responsive or recurrent cases
- Facial fold surgery is a significant alteration of conformation in show dogs

9　Scaling dermatoses frequently affect the face in many primary and secondary keratinisation defects (Figure 23.3).

10　The face is frequently affected in hypersensitivity dermatitis (Figure 23.4) although the specialised areas of the head (ears, muzzle and periorbital region) are usually the most severely affected. Common signs include:
- Face rubbing
- Cheilitis
- Preauricular erythema and alopecia

Table 23.2 Skin diseases which are localised to the face

Parasitic	
Infection	Feline pox virus
	Facial fold intertrigo
	Acute moist dermatitis in Rottweiler, Labrador and Golden Retrievers (Figure 23.2)
Hypersensitivity	Atopic dermatitis
	Adverse cutaneous reaction to food
Keratinisation defects	
Pigmentary changes	
Endocrine	
Nodular and granulomatous diseases	
Immune mediated	Angio-oedema, hives
Neoplasia	
Paraneoplastic syndromes	
Nutritional	
Miscellaneous	Facial pruritus of Persian cats
	Urticaria pigmentosa
	Snake, fly and spider bites

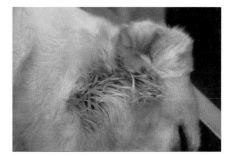

Figure 23.2 AMD lesion below the pinna of a Labrador Retriever.

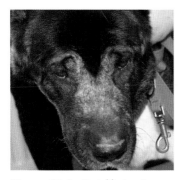

Figure 23.3 Facial lesions in an Akita with pemphigus foliaceus.

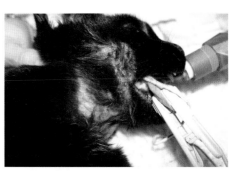

Figure 23.4 Preauricular eosinophilic plaques in cat with atopic dermatitis.

Chapter 24

Management of Skin Disease Affecting the Legs

Table 24.1 lists the diseases in which the legs are commonly involved.

Table 24.2 lists skin diseases which are commonly localised to the legs.

Figure 24.1 outlines the management of skin diseases affecting the legs. The numbers in the text refer to the numbers on the figure.

1 Skin lesions are most frequently found on the legs as part of a more generalised skin disease.

2 Skin lesions of the legs most frequently represent spread of conditions affecting the foot. In these cases the case should be investigated as in Chapter 18.3.

Table 24.1 Generalised skin diseases in which lesions occur on the legs

Parasitic	**Scabies**
	Trombiculosis
Infection	Feline TB
	Leprosy
	Pelodera
	FeLV dermatitis
	Rocky Mountain spotted fever
	Babesiosis
Hypersensitivity	**Atopic dermatitis**
	Cutaneous adverse reaction to food
	Parasitic hypersensitivity
Keratinisation defects	
Pigmentary changes	
Endocrine	
Nodular and granulomatous diseases	Feline TB
	Leprosy
Immune mediated	**Pemphigus complex**
	SLE
Neoplasia	Epitheliotrophic lymphoma
Paraneoplastic syndromes	Paraneoplastic pemphigus
	Necrolytic migratory erythema
Nutritional	
Miscellaneous	Vasculitis
	Feline pseudopelade
	Epidermolysis bullosa
	Familial canine dermatomyositis

Table 24.2 Skin diseases in which lesions are localised to the legs

Parasitic	
Infection	**Callus pyoderma**
Hypersensitivity	
Keratinisation defects	
Pigmentary changes	
Endocrine	
Nodular and granulomatous diseases	**Linear granuloma**
	Acral lick dermatitis
Immune mediated	
Neoplasia	Melanoma
	Haemangiopericytoma
Paraneoplastic syndromes	
Nutritional	
Miscellaneous	Snake and spider bites
	Metatarsal furunculosis of GSD
	Pressure sores
	Callus
	Hygroma
	Pododermatitis in Guinea pigs and rabbits

3 Raised nodular or ulcerative lesions should be biopsied early in the investigation (Figure 24.2).
   • Skin lesions restricted to the legs are less common, but there are several important diseases which should be investigated
   • Raised, nodular, erosive or ulcerated lesions should be investigated thoroughly and biopsy considered early on in the course of the disease to reach a definitive diagnosis
   • Feline TB and leprosy lesions are sometimes found on the leg
   • Haemangiopericytoma, while a benign neoplasm, frequently recurs and can be challenging to remove in an area with little free skin. Early diagnosis is essential
   • Pressure sores
     ◦ Pressure sores are an indicator of poor nursing
     ◦ Prevention is much easier than cure
     ◦ Caused by necrosis of deep soft tissues over bony prominence that erupt to surface
     ◦ Often complicated by maceration of tissues due to lying in body fluids and contamination
     ◦ Diligent nursing with regular turning
     ◦ More than adequately thick bedding materials
     ◦ Suitable bedding materials that wick away moisture
     ◦ Antibacterials to treat secondary infection
     ◦ Various substances have been used to accelerate healing
     ◦ Surgical closure may be necessary in severe cases
   • Pressure point callus/callus pyoderma
     ◦ Management problem in large breed dogs lying on hard surfaces (also sternum of Dachshunds)

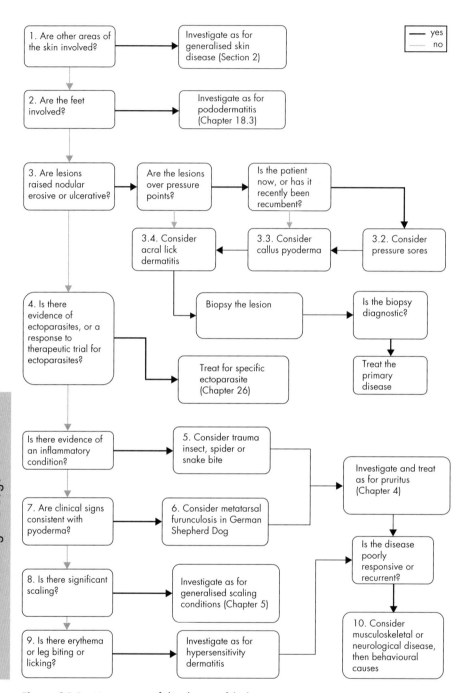

Figure 24.1   Management of skin disease of the legs.

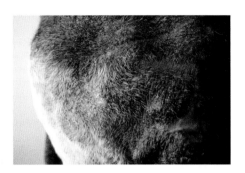

Figure 24.2 Telangiectasia is rare but has been reported to affect the shoulder and proximal forelimb.

- ○ Thickening of skin and hairloss usually only cosmetic
- ○ Resistant to treatment without correcting underlying cause
- ○ Cracked areas may respond to emollients and moisturisers
- ○ Furunculosis lesions may cause clinical problems
- ○ Address underlying cause
- ○ Topical antibiotic/steroid combinations
- ○ Systemic antibiotics
- ○ Tends to recur
- ○ Surgical excision not recommended as problems with wound healing
- ○ Occlusal dressings usually ineffective
- ○ Elbow hygromas are swellings of the elbow bursa caused by similar repeat friction (see Figure 2.18)
- • Acral lick lesions (Figure 24.3)
  - ○ Very challenging to treat
  - ○ Labrador Retrievers predisposed
  - ○ Many underlying causes including
  - ○ Demodicosis
  - ○ Dermatophytosis
  - ○ Hypersensitivity dermatitis

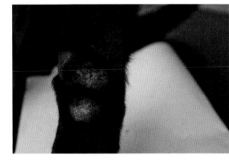

Figure 24.3 Acral lick dermatitis/furunculosis affecting the cranial carpus of a Labrador Retriever with hypersensitivity dermatitis.

- ◦ Musculoskeletal disease
- ◦ ? Behavioural
- ◦ Perpetuated by habituated licking
- ◦ Frequently becomes self-perpetuating due to self-trauma
- ◦ Histopathological lesion frequently one of furunculosis

Treatment

- Address the underlying cause, whether physical or behavioural
- Long-term glucocorticoid therapy (Chapter 28)
- Topical therapy should be used with caution to avoid increasing self-trauma (Chapter 29). DMSO may improve absorption if available
- Intralesional and parenteral glucocorticoids can also be considered (see Chapter 28)
- Behaviour modifying drugs
- Acupuncture
- Surgical excision usually unsuccessful because:
  - ◦ Lesions occur over bony prominences with firmly attached skin
  - ◦ Patient will not allow wound to heal unless primary cause addressed
  - ◦ Occlusal dressings usually result in temporary remission only
  - ◦ Cases where furunculosis identified need long courses of antibiotic therapy (see Chapter 27)

4 **Ectoparasites**
   - The legs are a predilection site for a number of parasites
     - ◦ *Neotrombicula autumnalis*
     - ◦ *Sarcoptes* spp.
     - ◦ Ticks

5 **Spider or snake bite, insect bite or sting**
   - The legs are a commonly affected site as animals disturb animals as they run through undergrowth

6 **Metatarsal furunculosis of German Shepherd Dog**
   Uncommon dermatosis of unknown aetiopathogenesis which appears to affect only the German Shepherd Dog. It resembles in appearance German Shepherd deep pyoderma and anal furunculosis and there may be a secondary bacterial furunculosis. However, the primary lesion is sterile and appears to be a collagen defect.

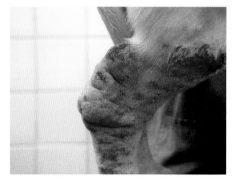

Figure 24.4 Severe hock lesions in deep pyoderma/furunculosis.

7 **Pyoderma** (Figure 24.4)
   - Pyoderma secondary to underlying primary disease is frequently found on the legs as part of a more generalised dermatitis, although infrequently in isolation

8 **Scaling** due to either primary or secondary keratinisation defect is frequently found on the legs as part of a more generalised dermatitis, although infrequently in isolation

9 **Erythema and pruritus** secondary to underlying hypersensitivity dermatitis is frequently found on the legs as part of a more generalised dermatitis, although infrequently in isolation (Figure 24.5)

10 **Other diseases resulting in self-trauma to the legs**
   These are usually a diagnosis of elimination. Skin disease should be ruled out before considering other causes:
   - Musculoskeletal disease may result in licking of painful areas
   - Self-mutilation may occur in neurological disease
   - Boredom, separation anxiety and habituation have been cited as causes of acral lick dermatitis, but physical causes must be ruled out first

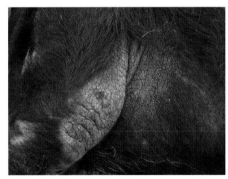

Figure 24.5 Axillary and proximal leg lesions in chronic inflammatory disease.

Chapter 25

Management of Diseases Affecting Mainly the Trunk and Dorsum

Figure 25.1 outlines the approach to diseases affecting the dorsum and trunk. The numbers in the text refer to the numbers on the figure.

Many dermatoses affect the trunk and dorsum of the patient as part of a more generalised problem, but a smaller number typically only affect this area. Tables 25.1 and 25.2 list the common causes of disease of the dorsum and trunk.

1 Ectoparasites
- Flea bite dermatitis commonly affects mainly the dorsum in both dogs and cats (Figure 25.2)
- Cheyletiellosis may present as dorsal scaling with or without pruritus
- Lesions caused by biting lice may be restricted to the dorsum although there is often a ventral papular rash or pyoderma
- Localised demodicosis lesions may occur anywhere including the dorsum, and the trunk is usually affected in generalised demodicosis

2 Dermatophytosis
- Dermatophytosis should always be considered in the presence of localised or generalised trunk lesions
- Fungal culture should always be performed in a cat with trunk lesions early in the investigation

3 Generalised skin disease
- A thorough history and clinical examination is essential to differentiate from generalised skin disease
- Secondary pyoderma and *Malassezia* dermatitis frequently affect the trunk and dorsum in generalised skin disease
- Dorsal scaling may frequently be seen in hypersensitivity dermatitis, sometimes as the only visible lesion in the West Highland White Terrier
- It is unusual for hypersensitivity dermatitis and other immune-mediated dermatoses to present with only dorsal or trunk lesions
- Zinc responsive dermatosis may present with dorsal scaling as one of many clinical signs

4 Systemic disease
- Truncal alopecia, dorsal scaling and secondary pyoderma are common early manifestations of systemic disease
- Skin signs may occur before systemic clinical signs
- Hypothyroidism and hyperadrenocorticism
- Diabetic dermatosis
- Paraneoplastic syndromes

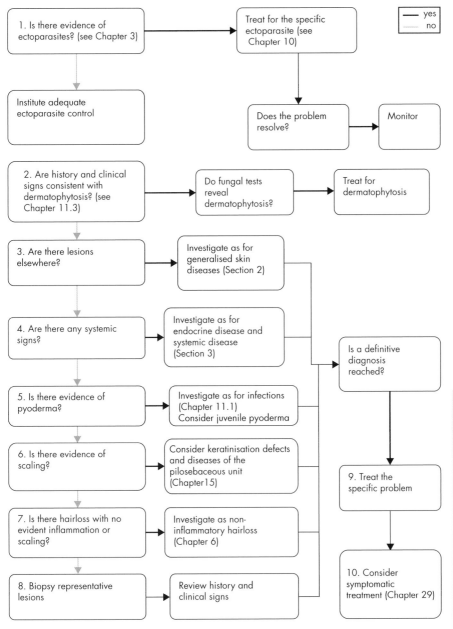

Figure 25.1   Management of diseases affecting the dorsum and trunk.

5   Pyoderma

- The ventral abdomen frequently demonstrates pustules due to pyoderma, which is usually secondary to an initiating cause
- In young animals ventral pyoderma may occur commonly in isolation and usually responds well to topical or, in more severe cases, systemic antibiotic treatment (see Chapter 27)

Table 25.1   Generalised diseases which often affect the dorsum and trunk

Ectoparasites	Flea bite dermatitis
	Cheyletiellosis
	Lice
	Demodicosis
	Scabies
	Ear mite dermatitis
Infection	Dermatophytosis
	Pyoderma
	Malassezia dermatitis
Hypersensitivity dermatitis	Contact irritant reaction
	Flea bite dermatitis
	Hypersensitivity dermatitis resulting in feline symmetrica alopecia in cats
Keratinisation defects	Primary keratinisation defect
	Secondary keratinisation defects especially in some breeds, for example, WHWT
Diseases of the pilosebaceous unit	Colour dilution alopecia
	Hair follicle dysplasias
	Sebaceous adenitis
	Congenital and hereditary alopecias
Endocrine disease	Hyperadrenocorticism
	Hypothyroidism
	Adrenal hyperplasia like syndrome (Alopecia X, adrenal sex hormone imbalance, growth hormone responsive dermatosis, castration responsive dermatosis), diabetic dermatosis
Non-endocrine alopecias	Recurrent symmetrical alopecia
	Congenital and hereditary alopecias
Immune-mediated disease	Pemphigus complex
Neoplastic	Many adnexal tumours
	Epitheliotrophic lymphoma
Paraneoplastic syndromes	Superficial necrolytic dermatitis (hepatocutaneous syndrome, metabolic epidermal necrosis, necrolytic migratory erythema)
Nutritional	Zinc responsive dermatosis
Miscellaneous	Trauma, burns and scalds

6   Diseases of the pilosebaceous unit frequently affect the dorsum and trunk, some are localised to the dorsum and trunk
- Some hair follicle dysplasias
- Sebaceous adenitis (Figure 25.3)

7   Non-inflammatory alopecia (Figures 25.4, 25.5)
- Non-inflammatory alopecias are frequently restricted to the dorsum and trunk
- Hereditary and congenital alopecias
- Endocrine alopecias frequently present with no other clinical signs

Table 25.2 Diseases which can be localised to the dorsum and trunk

Ectoparasites	Flea bite dermatitis
	Cheyletiellosis
	Lice
	Demodicosis
Infection	Dermatophytosis
	Juvenile superficial pyoderma
Hypersensitivity dermatitis	Contact irritant reaction
Keratinisation defects	Primary keratinisation defect
	Secondary keratinisation defect especially in some breeds, e.g. WHWT
Diseases of the pilosebaceous unit	Colour dilution alopecia
	Hair follicle dysplasias
	Sebaceous adenitis
Endocrine disease	Hyperadrenocorticism
	Hypothyroidism
	Adrenal hyperplasia-like syndrome (Alopecia X, adrenal sex hormone imbalance, growth hormone responsive dermatosis, castration responsive dermatosis)
Non-endocrine alopecias	Recurrent symmetrical alopecia
Immune-mediated disease	Pemphigus
	Erythema multiforme
Neoplastic	Many adnexal tumours
Miscellaneous	Trauma, burns and scalds

- Hyperadrenocorticism
- Hypothyroidism
- Adrenocortical dysplasia
- Non-endocrine alopecia
  - Seasonal flank alopecia is the most common non-endocrine alopecia normally associated with hairloss alone (Figure 25.4)
- Hair follicle dysplasias may present as a moth eaten appearance in the early stages but are more commonly associated with scaling

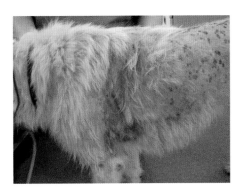

Figure 25.2 Erythema and excoriation due to self-trauma in a dog with flea bite dermatitis.

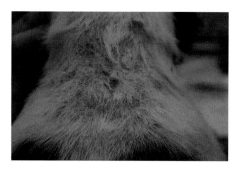

Figure 25.3 Dorsal scaling and hairloss in sebaceous adenitis.

8 Early biopsy of primary lesions

It may be difficult to distinguish primary lesions from secondary lesions with a similar appearance such as scaling and pyoderma but, if in doubt, early biopsy should be performed. Many conditions which usually affect the dorsum and trunk alone can be diagnosed by their histopathological changes.

Examples include:
• Hair follicle dysplasias
• Colour dilution alopecias
• Some paraneoplastic syndromes
• Neoplasia, including epitheliotrophic lymphoma
• Sebaceous adenitis

Biopsies may yield consistent information in many other dermatoses:
• *Malassezia* dermatitis
• Some immune-mediated diseases
• Endocrine skin disease
• Congenital and hereditary alopecias

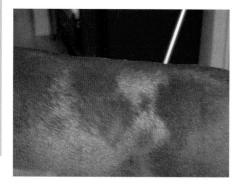

Figure 25.4 Bilateral flank alopecia in a boxer.

Management of Diseases Affecting
Mainly the Trunk and Dorsum

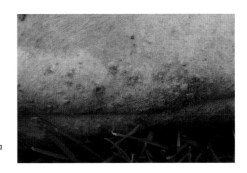

Figure 25.5 Ventral comedones in a Greyhound.

9   Specific treatments

Where there is a primary treatment available (see Chapter 26), these should be used, but supportive and topical treatments are often also necessary to control the condition.

10   Symptomatic treatment

There is no specific treatment for congenital and hereditary alopecias or hair follicle dysplasias. Although there are some primary treatments available for adrenal hyperplasia like syndrome (adrenal sex hormone imbalance, Alopecia X, growth hormone responsive dermatosis, castration responsive dermatosis) and seasonal flank alopecia, these are not always justified due to the systemic side-effects produced by drugs not licensed for the species treated in a disease which is largely cosmetic.

Scaling and pyoderma are common complications of these conditions and supportive and topical treatments are indicated (see Chapters 27 and 29). Psychogenic alopecia (Figure 25.6) is a controversial diagnosis of elimination. Environmental change or change in routine may lead to an improvement in signs.

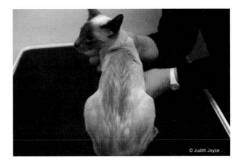

Figure 25.6 Dorsal hairloss in Siamese cat with suspected psychogenic alopecia.

SECTION 5

TREATMENT OF SKIN DISEASES

While every effort has been made to give accurate doses for the drugs used in treatments in this book, the veterinary surgeon should follow the current recommendations of the data sheet for any licensed products and the most up to date texts and literature for any product used off label.

Chapter 26

Treatment of Primary Skin Disease

26.1 ECTOPARASITICIDES

26.1.1 FLEAS

Control of fleas
Principles of flea control are detailed in Chapters 10.1.1, 10.2.1 and 10.3.1.

Adulticides
1. Rapid knock-down products followed by removal to clean environment
2. More frequently long-term effective control in the presence of the risk of reinfestation required

Use of adulticidal, insect growth regulators and physical methods
- There are many effective products for this purpose
- Topical products with residual action have largely superceded sprays, powders, shampoos and collars
- Frequent and regular use according to the manufacturers' requirements needed long term
- Especially when combined with insect growth regulators, environmental products not required in prevention of flea infestation
- In the face of flea infestation, environmental products desirable to reduce the flea burden within the house
  - Kill adult fleas in the house
  - Kill eggs and larvae by physical and chemical means
  - Insect growth regulators prevent development of fleas in the environment
- There are many effective flea control treatments on the market. Spot on preparations have largely taken the place of the messier, less well targeted sprays, powders and collars
- Fleas are well adapted parasites who only need the host species for a blood meal before egg laying. Can live independently of the host otherwise. Eggs, larvae and some adults live free in the environment
- Flea control is based on:
  - Adulticides and insect growth regulators targeting the patient
  - Adulticides and insect growth regulators targeting the environment
  - Some topical adulticides have some larvicidal effect

Common topical adulticides are listed in Table 26.1a.

Common insect growth regulators are listed in Table 26.1b.

Treatment of Primary Skin Disease

Table 26.1a Common flea adulticides in dogs and cats

Product	Formulation	Species	Dose duration and frequency	Contraindications	Adverse effects
Imidacloprid	Spot on	Dogs, cats and rabbits	400 mg/4 kg every 4 weeks	Animals less than 8 weeks old Rabbits for human consumption	Rare Local irritation
Imidacloprid and moxidextin	Spot on	Dogs and cats	Imidacloprid 10 mg/kg Moxidectin – cats 1 mg/kg Dogs 2.5 mg/kg monthly	Kittens less than 9 weeks Puppies less than 7 weeks Care under 1 kg BW Care in pregnancy and lactation	CNS signs Salivation due to bitter taste
Nitenpyram	Oral tablet	Dogs and cats	1 mg/kg daily when fleas are seen	Animals less than 4 weeks old Animals less than 1 kg	Generalised pruritus for 1 hour after application
Fipronil	Spot on	Dogs and cats	7.5–15 mg/kg every 4 weeks	Animals less than 8 weeks Cats less than 1 kg Dogs less than 2 kg Do not use in rabbits	Local irritation or pruritus Rare CNS signs Hypersalivation
Fipronil	Spray	Dogs and cats	7.5–15 mg/kg every 4 weeks	Do not use in rabbits Animals less than 2 days of age	Local irritation or generalised pruritus Rare CNS signs Hypersalivation
Fipronil with methoprene	Spot on	Dogs and cats	5 mg/kg fipronil 6 mg/kg methoprene Every 6 weeks	Do not use in rabbits Animals less than 8 weeks Cats less than 1 kg Dogs less than 2 kg	Local irritation or generalised pruritus Rare CNS signs Hypersalivation

Metaflumizone	Spot on	Cats	40 mg/kg every 6 weeks	Cats less than 8 weeks	Hypersalivation
Metaflumizone with amitraz	Spot on	Dogs	20 mg/kg metaflumizone 20 mg/kg amitraz every 4 weeks	Puppies under 8 weeks Do not use in cats	Hypersalivation CNS signs
Pyriprole	Spot on	Dogs	12.5 mg/kg monthly	Do not use in cats Do not use in rabbits Dogs less than 8 weeks old Dogs less than 2 kg	Hypersalivation Hypersensitivity reactions
Selamectin	Spot on	Dogs and cats	6 mg/kg every 4 weeks	Animals under 6 weeks	Transient localised hairloss
Imidacloprid with permethrin	Topical drops	Dogs	10 mg/kg imidacloprid 50 mg/kg permethrin every 4 weeks	Do not use on cats Puppies less than 7 weeks Dogs less than 1.5 kg	Transient local irritation Lethargy

Table 26.1b Commonly used insect growth regulators used in ectoparasite control

Product	Formulation	Species	Dose duration and frequency	Contraindications	Adverse effects
Lufenuron	Injection	Cats	10 mg/kg injected every 6 months	Do not use in dogs	
Lufenuron	Oral suspension	Cats	30 mg/kg monthly		
Lufenuron	Oral tablets	Dogs	10 mg/kg monthly		
Lufenuron + milbemycin	Oral tablets	Dogs	10 mg/kg lufenuron monthly		
Methoprene	Spot on with fipronil	Dogs and cats	6 mg/kg every 4–6 weeks	Do not use in rabbits Do not use in cats or dogs less than 8 weeks or 1 kg	Occasional pruritus after treatment Occasional hypersensitivity
Pyriproxifen	Environmental spray with permethrin	House	Yearly	Very toxic to fish Toxic to cats	
Cyromazine	Liquid pour on	Rabbits for flystrike	25 ml of 6% solution every 8–10 weeks	Rabbits less than 10 weeks old	Occasional inappetance
Dimeticone	Environmental spray	House	14 squirts per square metre every 6 weeks		May be slippery on hard surfaces when wet

26.1.2 SCABIES

- Treatment is based on the repeated use of acaricides beyond the length of the life cycle of the mite (3 weeks)
- Minimal environmental treatment is needed as all stages of the life cycle are found on the host
- Treat all in contact animals of same species
- Pruritus may persist well beyond the death of the mites due to hypersensitivity reactions to mite body parts and faeces. Adequate control of pruritus is essential to prevent potentiation of pruritic skin disease by self-trauma
- Pruritus associated with scabies is usually severe
- Drugs used commonly for the treatment of scabies are listed in Table 26.2

26.1.3 CHEYLETIELLA

- Treatment is based on repeated use of acaricides beyond the length of the life cycle of the mite (3 weeks)
- Treat all in contacts, may be cross infestation between dogs, cats and rabbits
- Pruritus is variable but antipruritics may be necessary

Table 26.2 Drugs used commonly for the treatment of scabies

Product	Formulation	Species	Dose duration and frequency	Contraindications	Adverse effects
Moxidectin/ imidacloprid	Spot on	Dogs and cats	Imidacloprid 10 mg/kg Moxidectin dogs 2.5 mg/kg Single treatment may be repeated after 4 weeks	Kittens less than 9 weeks Puppies less than 7 weeks Care under 1 kg BW Care in pregnancy and lactation	CNS signs Salivation due to bitter taste
Amitraz	Wash (not to be rinsed off)	Dogs	1 in 200 solution of 5% amitraz weekly for 2–6 weeks	Do not use in Chihuahuas Do not use in cats Puppies less than 3 months old Pregnant and lactating bitches	Sedation, lethargy CNS depression, bradycardia and slow shallow breathing Toxic to fish
Selamectin	Spot on	Dogs and cats	6 mg/kg single dose, may use extra dose after 30 days	Animals under 6 weeks	Transient localised hairloss

- Shampooing is always beneficial to remove excess scale, eggs and adult mites
- Bedding should be treated where possible. Washing followed by hot tumble drying is effective
- Environmental treatment with flea adulticides may be beneficial
- Drugs used commonly for the treatment of cheyletiellosis are listed in Table 26.3

26.1.4 EAR MITES

- *Otodectes cynotis* in dogs, cats, ferrets and hedgehogs
- *Psoroptes cuniculi* in rabbits
- Treatment is based on repeated use of adulticides beyond the life cycle of the mite (3 weeks) and physical removal of debris, mites and eggs
- Anaesthesia or sedation may be necessary in severe cases, especially for rabbits
- Do not use fipronil to treat rabbits
- Pruritus and discomfort are variable. Antipruritic treatments and pain relief should be used as necessary
- All in contact dogs, cats and ferrets must be treated
- Little environmental treatment necessary although some mites may be found on the hair coat outside the ear canal
- May cause hypersensitivity dermatitis in rare cases
- Drugs used commonly for the treatment of ear mites are listed in Table 26.4

Table 26.3 Drugs used in the treatment of cheyletiellosis

Product	Formulation	Species	Dose duration and frequency	Contraindications	Adverse effects
Moxidectin/ imidacloprid	Spot on	Dogs	Imidacloprid 10 mg/kg Moxidectin dogs 2.5 mg/kg Single treatment may be repeated after 4 weeks	Puppies less than 7 weeks Care under 1 kg BW Care in pregnancy and lactation	CNS signs Salivation due to bitter taste
Selamectin	Spot on	Dogs and cats	6 mg/kg single dose, may use extra dose after 30 days	Animals under 6 weeks	Transient localised hairloss
Fipronil	Spot on	Dogs and cats	7.5–15 mg/kg every 4 weeks	Rabbits, puppies and kittens under 8 weeks	Local pruritus, hypersalivation, rare CNS effects
Fipronil	Spray	Dogs and cats	7.5–15 mg/kg every 4 weeks	Rabbits, puppies and kittens under 2 days	Hypersalivation, rare CNS effects

Table 26.4 Drugs used commonly for the treatment of ear mites

Product	Formulation	Species	Dose duration and frequency	Contraindications	Adverse effects
Moxidectin/ imidacloprid	Spot on	Dogs and cats	Imidacloprid 10 mg/kg Moxidectin – cats 1 mg/kg Dogs 2.5 mg/kg Single treatment may be repeated after 4 weeks	Kittens less than 9 weeks Puppies less than 7 weeks Care under 1 kg BW Care in pregnancy and lactation	CNS signs Salivation due to bitter taste
Selamectin	Spot on	Dogs and cats	6 mg/kg single dose, may use an extra dose after 30 days	Animals under 6 weeks	Transient localised hairloss
Diethanolamine, framycetin, nystatin, prednisolone	Ear drops	Dogs and cats	Mode of action not known 5–10 drops twice daily	Perforated ear drums Pregnancy	Irritation May cause adrenocortical suppression

26.1.5 LICE

- Treatment based on use of acaricides beyond the life cycle of the louse (3 weeks)
- Treat all in contact animals of same species
- Fairly common in young puppies and working dogs
- Also found in debilitated pets due to lack of grooming
- Species specific
- Short survival away from host so environmental treatment not usually necessary
- The biting louse *Trichodectes canis* is much more common in dogs than the sucking louse, but most treatments used for the biting louse will be effective against the sucking louse
- Drugs used commonly for the treatment of lice are listed in Table 26.5

Table 26.5 Drugs used commonly for the treatment of biting lice

Product	Formulation	Species	Dose duration and frequency	Contraindications	Adverse effects
Moxidectin/ imidacloprid	Spot on	Dogs	Imidacloprid 10 mg/kg Moxidectin dogs 2.5 mg/kg Single treatment may be repeated after 4 weeks	Puppies less than 7 weeks Care under 1 kg BW Care in pregnancy and lactation	CNS signs Salivation due to bitter taste
Fipronil	Spot on	Dogs and cats	7.5–15 mg/kg every 4–8 weeks	Animals less than 8 weeks Cats less than 1 kg Dogs less than 2 kg Do not use in rabbits	Local irritation or pruritus Rare CNS signs Hypersalivation
Fipronil	Spray	Dogs and cats	7.5–15 mg/kg every 4–12 weeks	Do not use in rabbits Animals less than 2 days of age	Local irritation or generalised pruritus Rare CNS signs Hypersalivation
Fipronil with methoprene	Spot on	Dogs and cats	5 mg/kg fipronil 6 mg/kg methoprene Every 4–6 weeks	Animals less than 8 weeks old Cats less than 1 kg Dogs less than 2 kg	Local irritation or generalised pruritus Rare CNS signs Hypersalivation
Selamectin	Spot on	Dogs and cats	6 mg/kg single dose, may use extra dose after 30 days	Animals under 6 weeks	Transient localised hairloss

26.1.6 TICKS

- Ticks may cause problems in a number of ways:
  - Local irritation
  - Foreign body reaction following incomplete removal
  - As a vector of systemic disease, e.g. Lyme disease
- Ticks are frequently not noticed until they have been attached to the host for several days. Physical removal using a proprietary remover is usually adequate
- Insecticides mainly do not prevent the attachment of ticks but they are usually killed within 24 hours, which reduces transmission of disease and localised reaction. They usually fall off before the owner notices them
- Drugs used commonly for the treatment of ticks are listed in Table 26.6

26.1.7 DEMODICOSIS

- Common in young dogs of short haired breeds
- Can occur spontaneously or as a result of immunosuppressive disease in mature animals (especially American Cockers Spaniel and West Highland White Terrier)
- Aggressive management is always essential
- **Pododemodicosis is especially challenging to diagnose and treat**
- Find the mite by scrapings and perform live:dead ratio count
- Where deep skin scrapes are negative and demodicosis is still suspected, biopsy representative lesions
- Investigate underlying immunosuppressive causes where appropriate
- Clip long hair coats before treatment
- Pre-wash with 'follicle flushing shampoo' (e.g. benzoyl peroxide) before each treatment
- Use fresh amitraz exactly according to manufacturer's instructions
- Repeat live:dead ratio counts every 4 weeks
- Continue with treatments 4 weeks beyond all dead or all gone
- Concurrent systemic antibacterial therapy essential
- Choose appropriate antibiotic at correct dose, continue beyond 'cure'
- The use of glucocorticoids in any case of demodicosis is always contraindicated
- Pain relief should be considered
- Drugs used commonly for the treatment of demodicosis are listed in Table 26.7

Although there are many reports of the use of avermectins in demodicosis, their use is off label for this purpose and there are safety concerns regarding their use at the high doses necessary.

High dose oral or injected avermectin regimens are indicated in particularly severe and treatment resistant cases of demodicosis, particularly pododemodicosis, where euthanasia may be the only other appropriate treatment option.

Milbemycin oxime at a dose rate of 0.5–1.2 mg/kg once daily for 2–3 months has been reported to be effective.

Some individuals of a number of breeds including rough and smooth collies and some sighthounds have mdr1 gene deletion which results in toxicity. The off label use of avermectins is contraindicated in these individuals or in these breeds if gene testing is not available.

Table 26.6 Drugs used commonly for the treatment of ticks

Product	Formulation	Species	Dose duration and frequency	Contraindications	Adverse effects
Fipronil	Spot on	Dogs and cats	7.5–15 mg/kg every 4 weeks	Animals less than 8 weeks Cats less than 1 kg Dogs less than 2 kg Do not use in rabbits	Local irritation or pruritus Rare CNS signs Hypersalivation
Fipronil	Spray	Dogs and cats	7.5–15 mg/kg every 4 weeks	Do not use in rabbits Animals less than 2 days of age	Local irritation or generalised pruritus Rare CNS signs Hypersalivation
Fipronil with methoprene	Spot on	Dogs and cats	5 mg/kg fipronil 6 mg/kg methoprene Every 4 weeks	Do not use in rabbits Animals less than 8 weeks Cats less than 1 kg Dogs less than 2 kg	Local irritation or generalised pruritus Rare CNS signs Hypersalivation
Metaflumizone combined with amitraz	Spot on	Dogs	20 mg/kg metaflumizone 20 mg/kg amitraz every 4 weeks	Puppies under 8 weeks Do not use in cats	Hypersalivation CNS signs
Pyriprole	Spot on	Dogs	12.5 mg/kg monthly	Do not use in cats Do not use in rabbits Dogs less than 8 weeks old Dogs less than 2 kg	Hypersalivation Hypersensitivity reactions
Deltamethrin	Collar	Dogs	0.76–1 g per collar Every 5–6 months	Do not use on cats Do not use with other organophosphate products Puppies less than 7 weeks Dogs with skin lesions	CNS signs if collar eaten
Imidacloprid with permethrin	Topical drops	Dogs	10 mg/kg imidacloprid 50 mg/kg permethrin every 4 weeks	Do not use on cats Puppies less than 7 weeks Dogs less than 1.5 kg	Transient local irritation Lethargy
Selamectin (not effective against *Ixodes ricinus*)	Spot on	Dogs and cats	6 mg/kg single dose, monthly	Animals under 6 weeks	Transient localised hairloss

Table 26.7 Drugs commonly used and licensed for the primary treatment of demodicosis

Product	Formulation	Species	Dose duration and frequency	Contraindications	Adverse effects
Amitraz	Wash (not to be rinsed off)	Dogs	1 in 100 solution of 5% amitraz every 5–7 days 3 weeks beyond clinical cure +negative skin scrapes	Do not use in Chihuahuas Do not use in cats Puppies less than 3 months old Pregnant and lactating bitches	Sedation, lethargy CNS depression, bradycardia and slow shallow breathing Toxic to fish
Imidacloprid and moxidextin	Spot on	Dogs and cats	Imidacloprid 10 mg/kg Moxidectin – cats 1 mg/kg Dogs 2.5 mg/kg monthly	Kittens less than 9 weeks Puppies less than 7 weeks Care under 1 kg BW Care in pregnancy and lactation	CNS signs Salivation due to bitter taste

The advice of the drug company should be sought before these products are used and the owners made aware of safety concerns before use so that they can give informed consent.

26.1.8 HARVEST MITES

- Harvest mites favour alkaline soils. Not all stages of the life cycle are parasitic but irritation due to their bites occurs commonly in some areas
- Diagnosis is often challenging as the mite may have returned to the environment before clinical signs of hypersensitivity are noted
- Face, ears and feet are commonly affected and the mites are visible to the naked eye
- There are no licensed treatments for harvest mites but fipronil spray has been used with success in some cases

26.1.9 FLIES

- Flies may cause disease in a number of ways:
  - Irritant reaction
  - Hypersensitivity reaction
  - Transmission of disease, e.g. leishmaniasis
  - Fly strike
- Treatment is based on keeping animals away from areas where flies are prevalent, for example, humid still environments, early morning and late evening walks, macerated tissues
- Chemical repellents and killers may also be used. Topical cyromazine is licensed for use in rabbits at risk of fly strike
- Drugs used for this purpose are listed in Table 26.8

Treatment of Primary Skin Disease

Table 26.8 Drugs commonly used to repel or kill flies

Product	Formulation	Species	Dose duration and frequency	Contraindications	Adverse effects
Imidacloprid with permethrin	Topical drops	Dogs	10 mg/kg imidacloprid 50 mg/kg permethrin every 4 weeks	Do not use in cats Puppies less than 7 weeks Dogs less than 1.5 kg	Transient local irritation Lethargy
Deltamethrin	Collar	Dogs	0.76–1 g per collar Every 5–6 months	Do not use in cats Do not use with other organophosphate products Puppies less than 7 weeks Dogs with skin lesions	CNS signs if collar eaten
Cyromazine	Liquid pour on	Rabbits for flystrike	25 ml of 6% solution every 8–10 weeks	Rabbits less than 10 weeks old	Occasional inappetance

26.1.10 ECTOPARASITES OF SMALLER MAMMALS

Table 26.9 lists products used commonly for the treatment of ectoparasites in smaller mammals.

Many treatments have been used for the treatment of ectoparasites in the smaller mammals. However, these treatments are often off label and advice should be sought from the manufacturer before using them in each individual case.

26.2 TREATMENT OF DISEASES CAUSED BY MICRO-ORGANISMS

26.2.1 TREATMENT OF FUNGAL AND YEAST DISEASE

Dermatophytosis
- A primary fungal infection in a number of pet species caused by a number of fungi which have a specific tropism for keratin containing structures
- Can become a major problem in cat colonies
- Prompt diagnosis and treatment essential because of zoonotic potential
- Owners should be warned, especially regarding immune compromised or diabetic in contact humans
- Active spores may remain in environment for considerable lengths of time

Principles of treatment
- Identify and address the source of the infection (e.g. new kittens in the house)
- Treat the whole in contact group
- Monitor treatment with repeat fungal cultures
- Continue treatment beyond negative fungal culture

Treatment of Primary Skin Disease

Table 26.9 Ectoparasiticides of smaller mammals (and other animals)

Product	Formulation	Indications	Species	Dose duration frequency	Contraindications	Adverse effects
Permethrin	Topical drops	Fleas Fly strike Ticks Lice	Rabbit, guinea pig, rat, hamster, chinchilla, mice other small rodents, birds	50 μg /250 g every 2 weeks	Very toxic to cats Animals under 16 weeks Ferrets Pregnant and lactating animals	CNS disturbances in rodents Extremely dangerous to fish Local irritation and lesions
Ivermectin	Spray	Mite infestations	Rabbits, guinea pigs, ferrets Small rodents Reptiles and birds	400 μg/kg 200 μg/kg 200 μg/kg monthly for prevention 0, 2 and 4 weeks for treatment	Animals less than 100 g Animals under 16 weeks Chelonians Pregnant and lactating animals	CNS signs Lethargy and inappetance Local irritation
Ivermectin	Topical drops	Mite infestations	Rats, mice, gerbils, chinchillas, hamsters, other rodents. Rabbits, ferrets and guinea pigs Birds	200–400μg/kg	Other species Pregnant and lactating animals Animals under 16 weeks Chelonians	CNS signs Lethargy and inappetance Local irritation
Imidacloprid	Topical drops	Fleas	Rabbits	400 mg/4 kg Up to weekly	Rabbits less than 10 weeks old Rabbits for human consumption	Rare Local irritation
Selamectin	Topical drops	Fleas, mite infestations	Off label Rabbits, ferrets, guinea pigs, hedgehogs, etc.	6 mg/kg every 4 weeks		
Amitraz	Wash	Mite infestations	Off label Rabbits, ferrets, guinea pigs, hedgehogs, etc.			
Fipronil	Topical drops	Fleas, ticks	Off label Ferrets, hedgehogs		Do not use in rabbits	
Cyromazine	Liquid pour on	Fly strike	Rabbits	25 ml of 6% solution every 8–10 weeks	Rabbits less than 10 weeks old	Occasional inappetance

- Carrier status in cat colonies is controversial but may remain a reservoir of infection
- Usually combination treatment necessary

Systemic treatments
Itraconazole

Formulation
- Oral liquid

Mode of action
- High affinity for fungal cytochrome P-450, effective at doses which should not affect mammalian cytochrome P-450
- Inhibits cytochrome P-450 demethylase, reducing synthesis of ergosterol, which is essential for maintaining fungal cell wall

Indications
- Dermatophytosis in cats
- Off label use for dermatophytosis in dogs, rodents and lagomorphs
- Off label use for *Malassezia* dermatitis and otitis externa in dogs and cats

Dose
- 5 mg/kg daily for 3 alternate weeks, that is:

Week 1	Week 2	Week 3	Week 4	Week 5
Daily dosing at 5 mg/kg	No dosing	Daily dosing at 5 mg/kg	No dosing	Daily dosing at 5 mg/kg

- Can be given directly into mouth before food once daily
- Can be given with a small amount of food to aid dosing
- Other regimens have been used for *Malassezia* dermatitis, e.g. daily dosing at 5 mg/kg for 3 weeks
- >90% efficacy in cats
- More effective than griseofulvin
- Well tolerated in young kittens

Contraindications
- Care in pregnant and lactating queens
- Care in impaired liver function

Adverse reactions
- Transient salivation, vomiting and diarrhoea, as well as blood biochemistry changes have been noted at 3–5 times of normal dose
- No major drug interactions have been noted, but care required with concomitant use of cyclosporin, rifampicin, phenobarbitone, digoxin or methylprednisolone or prednisolone

Safety information
Care with handling

Griseofulvin
The use of this drug is now probably contraindicated in view of its teratogenicity in the presence of a safer alternative. The drug is not licensed for this use in dogs and cats nor the smaller mammals.

Formulation
- 125 and 500 mg tablets

Mode of action
- Stops fungal cells dividing

Indication
- Off label use for dermatophytosis in several species

Dose
- 20 mg/kg once daily for at least 3 weeks but beyond negative culture

Contraindications
- Pregnancy, lactation breeding stock
- Young animals

Adverse effects
- Teratogenicity
- Bone marrow suppression
- Hepatopathy
- Gastrointestinal effects

Safety information
- This drug should not be handled by women of child bearing potential
- Owners should be given this information in writing

Topical treatments
Enilconazole

Formulation
- Topical rinse supplied in concentrated form of 100 mg/ml

Mode of action
- Inhibition of fungal cytochrome P-450 dependent 14a methylation of lanosterol ergosterol, component of membrane

Indication
- Dermatophytosis in several species, but not cats
- Other fungal infections

Dose
- Dilute 1 in 50 and use as a rinse, leaving on
- Clip long haired coats
- Repeat 4 times every 3 days

Contraindications
- Cats
- For external use only

Adverse effects
- None on data sheet

Safety information
- Wear protective clothing
- Dispose of leftover wash carefully

Miconazole/chlorhexidine shampoo
Formulation
- Shampoo containing 2% chlorhexidine and 2% miconazole

Mode of action
- Inhibits cell wall synthesis

Indication
- An adjunctive treatment for dermatophytosis in cats and dogs

Dose
- Shampoo twice weekly for 4–6 weeks minimum or until negative fungal culture is achieved
- Leave on for 10 minutes to allow sufficient contact time and rinse off well

Contraindications
- Cats may be non-compliant
- Nursing females unless puppies or kittens can be kept away until the coat is dry
- Do not allow the patient to lick
- Should only be used in conjunction with griseofulvin in cats
- For external use only

Adverse effects
- None reported on data sheet

Safety information
- Wear gloves, can dry hands
- Sensitivity to chlorhexidine can occur
- Care is always necessary when bathing cats

Environmental treatment
- Vacuuming
- Disinfection of grooming tools, toys, etc. Enilconazole can be used for this purpose in canine dermatophytosis, but care should be exercised when items may come in contact with cats
- Many other disinfectants have antifungal actions
- Clipped off and groomed out hair and debris should be disposed of straight away

Malassezia dermatitis
Principles of treatment
- Usually secondary, so it is important to address the primary cause
- May be more resistant to treatment if hypersensitivity reaction to *Malassezia* occurs
- But it is too early to give results for efficacy
- Topical treatments are usually sufficient, but systemic treatments may be indicated in hypersensitivity, resistant cases or where the primary cause cannot be identified or addressed

Topical treatments
Chlorhexidine/miconazole shampoo
- As above

Enilconazole
- As above
- Do not use in cats

Systemic treatments
Itraconazole
- As above, but off label use

Ketoconazole
Formulation
- 100 mg tablets

Mode of action
- Inhibition of ergosterol synthesis, important in fungal cell membrane structure

Indication
- Off label treatment of *Malassezia* dermatitis resistant to topical treatments
- It has also been used for other fungal infections

Dose
- 5 mg/kg daily in divided doses until resolution of signs

Contraindications
- Pregnant or lactating animals
- Ketoconazole reacts adversely with a number of other drugs, so care should be taken when the patient is on other drugs and advice sought
- There may be other unknown contraindications as this drug is used off label

Adverse effects
- Hepatotoxicity
- Cardiovascular effects, especially with some drug combinations
- There may be other unknown adverse effects as this drug is used off label

Safety information
- Owners should avoid handling the drug directly

Allergen specific immunotherapy
Patients with positive serological tests to *Malassezia* may benefit from *allergen specific immunotherapy* (ASIT, see Chapter 26.3)

Bacterial infections
Most bacterial infections are secondary to an underlying primary cause or predisposing factors. For this reason, **the treatment of bacterial infections is outlined in Chapter 27.2.**

Viruses
Primary treatment
- For most viral diseases supportive treatment alone is either adequate or all that is available

Interferon
Formulation
- Powder and solvent for suspension for injection

Mode of action
- Inhibition of the synthesis mechanisms of the infected cell, reducing viral replication

Indications
- Off label for feline respiratory viruses

Dose
- Dogs 2.5 million units (MU)/kg intravenously once daily for 3 days
- Cats 1 MU/kg intravenously once daily for 5 days 3 times starting on days 1, 14 and 60

Contraindications
- Concurrent vaccination
- Care should be taken in the presence of systemic illness
- No data on use in pregnant and lactating animals

Adverse effects
- Efficacy is dependent on adherence to dosing schedule

Safety information
- Dispose of left over product safely

Supportive treatments
- Although viral papillomatosis will resolve with time, surgical removal or debridement may be necessary if the presence of the masses compromises function or results in discomfort, secondary bacterial infection or bleeding
- Vaccination in the face of an outbreak may be indicated, e.g. rabbit myxomatosis
- Control of vectors of disease is usually indicated, e.g. control of exposure to the rabbit flea in myxomatosis
- Nursing of systemically ill patients greatly improves prognosis

Leishmaniasis
Principles of treatment
- Euthanasia should be considered in these cases due to their zoonotic potential
- As there are no veterinary licensed treatments for this condition all primary treatments should be used with caution
- Supportive treatments are beneficial and will improve prognosis

Primary treatments
Advice should be sought before using these treatments on an individual case basis as their use is off label.

- Meglumine antimoniate minimum dose of 100 mg/kg daily for at least 3–4 weeks, combined with allopurinol to reduce relapse rate
- Pentamidine – 4 mg/kg twice weekly
- Aminosidine 5 mg/kg twice daily for 3–4 weeks
- There is little evidence to support the use of some of the other treatments which have been suggested including allopurinol alone, amphotericin B, ketoconazole, enrofloxacin or metronidazole combined with enrofloxacin or spiramycin

Supportive treatments
- Cutaneous leishmaniasis is one manifestation of the disease and disease due to systemic signs should be addressed
- Control secondary pyoderma

Treatment of Primary Skin Disease

- Shampooing may be beneficial depending on clinical signs
- Deltamethrin collars and spot on permethrin are useful as fly repellents
- Avoid sand fly areas and times of day (late afternoon) as far as possible

26.3 TREATMENT OF HYPERSENSITIVITY DERMATITIS

Long-term control of hypersensitivity dermatitis can be frustrating

1. Constant review of underlying diagnosis.
- Flare factors exacerbate pruritus
- Concomitant disease
  - Atopic dogs are more likely to suffer from flea bite dermatitis
  - New hypersensitivities may develop
  - Other pruritic disease may develop
- Complications of treatment
  - Long-term use of glucocorticoids may increase risk of bacterial, yeast and fungal infections, e.g. demodicosis in West Highland White Terrier
  - Long-term use of glucocorticoids may result in dry hair coat, hairloss and scaling
  - Long-term use of cyclosporin may suppress immune system

2. Hypersensitivity dermatitis tends to become more severe and refractory to treatment with time.

- Increased number of allergens reacted to:
- Chronic change in the skin results in worsening of flare factors and secondary complications
- Chronic changes in skin being less amenable to treatment

3. There is now evidence that one of the primary defects in hypersensitivity dermatitis is an impaired epidermal barrier.

This allows the transmission of antigens and micro-organisms to the dermis. Longstanding pruritus, erythema and self-trauma damaging the physical and chemical structure of the skin exacerbate this.

4. Hypersensitivity dermatitis may become self-perpetuating. There is also now some evidence that with time atopic dermatitis no longer needs an external trigger and becomes self-perpetuating. Avoidance of allergens and ASIT therefore become less effective.

5. Treatments can be targeted as follows:

Damage to the epidermal barrier
- Prevent further damage by control of pruritus (see Chapter 27.1)
- Supplement the epidermal barrier with essential fatty acid and cofactor containing supplements and foods (see Chapter 27.1)
- Essential fatty acid containing shampoos (see Chapter 27.1)
- Address the primary disease

Control the clinical signs of hypersensitivity dermatitis
- Avoidance

- Immunomodulation
- Drug control

Parasite hypersensitivity
- **Avoidance** is the treatment of choice
- Ectoparasitic treatment is listed in Chapter 26.1
- **Immunomodulation** has been used in flea bite dermatitis but is generally unsuccessful
- **Drug control** is often necessary for support in the short term and in some cases of flea bite dermatitis in the long term
  - Control pruritus (Chapter 27.1)
  - Control secondary pyoderma and scaling (Chapters 27.2 and 27.3)
  - Nutritional support of skin (see Chapter 27.4)

Adverse cutaneous reaction to food
- **Avoidance** is the treatment of choice
- Select a diet which does not contain the allergens long term
- Feed hydrolysed diet long term
- Diets with restricted protein sources may be trialled, but may contain traces of other feedstuffs which may result in failure of treatment
- **Immunomodulation** has been attempted but is generally unsuccessful

Secondary effects on coat condition and scaling
- Essential fatty acids
- Chinese herbal supplements
- Shampoos and topical treatments
- **Drug control** is often necessary for support in the short term. Where poor compliance of adverse cutaneous reaction to food is one of several reactions (e.g. concurrent atopic dermatitis), long-term drug control is usually necessary.
  - Control pruritus (Chapter 27.1)
  - Control secondary pyoderma and scaling (Chapters 27.2 and 27.3)
  - Nutritional support of skin (see Chapter 27.4)

Atopic dermatitis
- **Avoidance** is rarely achievable
- Some epidermal allergens and house dust mite avoidance can be achieved by outdoor kennelling
- Reports of house dust mite control using boric acid powders alone in some European countries
- Reducing exposure to house dust mite is rarely sufficient to control the problem but may reduce clinical signs and hence reduce the need for long-term drug therapy
  - Outdoor kennelling of the pet where practical
  - Restrict the pet to kitchen and hard-surfaced areas
  - No access to bed and bathrooms where house dust mite populations are higher
  - Acaricidal sprays – some environmental flea sprays now have an indication for house dust mite. Active chemicals include permethrin and benzyl benzoate
  - Dehydrating powders, such as boric acid
  - Hot washing, tumble drying and freezing of pet bedding

- ○ Encasing bedding in plastic
- ○ Infrequent damp dusting
- ○ Hoovers adapted for reduced 'exhaust'
- ○ Avoiding the environment which the house dust mite favours, i.e. 25°C and 80% humidity – rarely acceptable to other inhabitants of the house who favour similar conditions
- ○ Prolonged periods of relative humidity less than 50% result in mite desiccation
- ○ Insect growth regulators are only effective in reducing mite population for about 1 month

Many human allergy websites can offer valuable advice on reducing exposure to house dust mite

Immunomodulation
Allergen specific immunotherapy (ASIT)

- Following a confirmed diagnosis of atopic dermatitis based on history and clinical signs, identification of allergens for ASIT can be made using intradermal test or serology (Chapter 3).
- **There is no licensed ASIT in the UK.**
- Allergen combinations for subcutaneous injection can be obtained from the Netherlands under a Special Import Certificate issued from the VMD.
- Allergen combinations from the USA can be obtained under a Special Treatment Certificate issued from the VMD.
- It is not known exactly how ASIT works although theories include antibody blocking and exhausting the antigenic receptors on cells.
- Reported success rates vary significantly from rare reports of nearly 100% in the USA to 40% in the UK. This may be due to the higher incidence of house dust mite hypersensitivity in the UK.
- Cases in which even a moderate response is seen (approximately 2/3 cases) may benefit from continued ASIT as long-term drug therapy can be reduced in these cases.
- Response time is slow – on average 5 months after the initiation of treatment. However, up to 9 months may elapse before optimum response is seen and some studies have suggested that even longer duration of treatment (up to 18 months) are necessary in some cases. Work is being conducted on faster induction protocols to try to achieve more rapid response.
- Long-term or lifelong therapy is usually needed although the frequency of administration can be reduced in some cases.
- Response to ASIT following intradermal testing and the more advanced serological tests appear to yield similar results.
- Immunosuppressive treatments should be avoided during the loading phase of treatment as far as patient comfort allows.
- There is some evidence that the efficacy in young patients who are treated soon after diagnosis is better than in chronic atopic dermatitis.
- There is some evidence that there may be more relapse in patients where ASIT is started at less than 1 year of age as the patient may become reactive to more allergens in the future. In these cases retesting should be considered.
- Relapse frequently occurs due to the presence of flare factors.
- Although there is much less information about atopic dermatitis and ASIT in cats, results appear to be similar.

Bacterial, yeast and fungal hypersensitivity
- Elimination
- ASIT
- Bacterial products

Flare factors
- These should be considered initially then reviewed and addressed on a regular basis.

Concurrent other diseases
- Ectoparasitic disease
- Secondary demodicosis for patients on long term immunosuppressive treatment
- Secondary yeast infections
- Dermatophytosis

Secondary pyoderma
- Long-term use of immunosuppressive treatments
- Chronically inflamed skin
- Damage to physical, chemical and immunological barriers of skin, both primary and secondary

Pruritic effects of build up on the skin
- Scale
- Grease
- Sweat
- Irritant products of inflammation
- Bacteria and yeasts

It is likely that the use of long-term therapy is necessary in cases of hypersensitivity dermatitis. The following should be considered when choosing the treatment for the patient.

- Evidence for efficacy
- Side-effects, both in short- and long-term use
- Label restrictions
- Ease of administration
- Drug interactions
- Cost

See Chapters 27.1 and 28 for details of these drugs and their use.

See Chapter 29 for details of topical treatments which may be useful adjunctive treatments in hypersensitivity dermatitis.

26.4 TREATMENT OF IMMUNE-MEDIATED DISEASE

It is important to avoid doing unnecessary harm in the treatment of immune-mediated disease by reserving drugs with side-effects for the most severe diseases and those where response to conservative treatment is poor.

- Many immune-mediated diseases are mild
- It is difficult to make a definitive diagnosis in many cases of suspected immune-mediated disease

- If trigger factors are addressed clinical signs may resolve spontaneously or with supportive treatment only
- The immune-mediated signs may only be part of the clinical picture

Primary treatment
- Identify and remove trigger factors where possible
- Investigate disease affecting other organ systems
- Immunosuppressive treatment based on glucocorticoids and other immunomodulating drugs should be reserved for more severe cases

Supporting treatment
- Pain relief should be considered
- Treat secondary bacterial, yeast and fungal infections
- Treat scaling and coat condition to improve patient comfort and reduce secondary infections

Topical treatment
- Shampooing always beneficial when not too painful
  - Treat secondary infectious disease
  - Remove scale and debris
  - Increase patient comfort
  - Improve absorption of topical treatments
- Topical treatments alone may be sufficient in mild immune-mediated disease
- Topical treatments alone of localised lesions preferable to avoid unnecessary drug side-effects

26.4.1   PRIMARY TREATMENTS OF IMMUNE-MEDIATED DISEASE

Supporting treatments for these conditions are detailed in Chapter 27.

CONSERVATIVE TREATMENTS

Topical treatment alone
- Suitable for discrete lesions
- Sunscreens are often indicated as immune-mediated disease is often exacerbated by exposure to sunlight

Topical glucocorticoids
Formulation
- Creams, ointments, gels and sprays

Mode of action
- Gene repression of multiple transcription factors for cytokines and their receptors, chemotactic proteins, adhesion molecules and pro-inflammatory enzymes
- Prevents the activation of many immune cells, e.g. T cells, eosinophils, macrophages and dendritic cells
- Can also activate anti-inflammatory genes
- Vehicles are usually emollient

Treatment of Primary Skin Disease

Indications
- As sole treatment in mild disease such as discoid lupus erythematosis
- As a palliative adjunct in discrete lesions of more severe disease

Dose
- According to manufacturer's instructions

Contraindications
- Care should be taken in the use of topical steroid treatment in dogs with diabetes mellitus and hyperadrenocorticism
- Deep pyoderma and some cases of superficial pyoderma
- In areas which are readily licked which will exacerbate the condition
- More extensively affected areas
- More severe immune-mediated disease where application may be painful
- Pregnancy

Adverse effects
- Many topical glucocorticoids suppress adrenal function
- Other steroid side-effects
- Self-trauma

Safety information
- Owners should wear gloves to use these preparations
- Patients should be deterred from licking

Tacrolimus ointment
- This has been used as an anti-inflammatory agent off label in a number of conditions. However, there are safety concerns for the owner in handling this compound and its use in pets is therefore controversial.

Nutritional support
- These are normally used as adjunctive therapy but occasionally as the primary treatment in mild immune-mediated disease
- Vitamin E
- Essential fatty acids
- Zinc

Niacinamide and tetracycline
Formulation
- Tablets and capsules

Mode of action
- Both have been shown to suppress various inflammatory pathways and antibody production

Indications
- Mild to moderate immune-mediated disease

Dose
- Dogs less than 10 kg, 250 mg of niacinamide and 250 mg tetracycline 3 times daily for a minimum of 2 weeks
- Dogs over 10 kg, 500 mg of niacinamide and 500 mg tetracycline 3 times daily for a minimum of 2 weeks

Contraindications
- As this is an off label use of both drugs, care should be taken in their usage
- Pregnancy and lactation

Adverse effects
- Gastrointestinal effects occasionally reported
- Hepatopathy and blood dyscrasias have been reported

Safety information
- General precautions

MORE AGGRESSIVE TREATMENTS

Glucocorticoids
- Prednisolone is the most commonly used oral preparation, but others such as triamcinolone have also been used
- The use and abuse of glucocorticoid preparations is detailed in Chapter 28
- Depot preparations should not be used

Formulation
- Oral tablets

Mode of action
- Gene repression of multiple transcription factors for cytokines and their receptors, chemotactic proteins, adhesion molecules and pro-inflammatory enzymes
- Prevents the activation of many immune cells, e.g. T cells, eosinophils, macrophages and dendritic cells
- Can also activate anti-inflammatory genes

Indications
- Moderate to severe cases of immune-mediated disease as first line treatment
- Non-responsive cases of mild to moderate immune-mediated disease

Dose
- Mild to moderate disease – dogs 1–2 mg/kg; cats 1–3 mg/kg
- Moderate to severe disease – immunosuppressive doses – dogs 2–4 mg/kg; cats 3–6 mg/kg
- Where a trigger factor can be identified and addressed short courses of 6 weeks may be sufficient
- Where a trigger factor cannot be identified, treatment should be withdrawn gradually after 6 weeks and again after 6 months to 'test' for resolution
- After initial treatment for 6 weeks, alternate day dosing should be initiated and the lowest possible maintenance dose achieved (see Chapter 28)

Contraindications
- Diabetes mellitus
- Demodicosis
- Dermatophytosis
- Immunosuppressive disease
- Neoplasia

Adverse effects
- As these are dose dependent, these are more common and more severe at immunosuppressive doses

- Polydypsia/polyuria
- Polyphagia and scavenging
- Muscle, tendon and ligament weakening
- Hyperadrenocorticism
- Diabetes mellitus
- Pancreatitis
- Hepatolipidosis
- Secondary urinary tract infections

Safety information
- Some patients may be depressed or show changes in behaviour on glucocorticoids

Azathioprine
Formulation
- Tablets

Mode of action
- Azathioprine is converted to a purine antagonist and inhibits DNA synthesis in activated lymphocytes

Indications
- This is an off label use of this drug, so it should be reserved for more severe and non-responsive immune-mediated disease. It is frequently used concomitantly with prednisolone to reduce the dose of steroid necessary.

Dose
- 1 mg/kg once daily initially, reducing the dose as necessary to maintenance levels after 4–6 weeks

Contraindications
- Cats
- Pregnancy
- Neoplasia

Adverse effects
- Hepatopathy
- Bone marrow suppression and reduced circulating blood cells
- Susceptibility to infections and possibly neoplasia
- Gastrointestinal disorders

Safety information
- Owners should not come into direct contact with the tablets

Cyclosporin
Formulation
Capsules

Indications for use
- Off label use for immune moderate to severe immune-mediated disease but data to support its use
- May be used off label concomitantly with prednisolone to reduce the dose of steroid required

Mode of action
- T cell activation inhibitor
- T cell cytokine inhibitor
- Mast cell inhibitor
- Reduced eosinophil survival

Dose
- Initial dose of 5 mg/kg daily, reducing to 5 mg/kg every other day after 6 weeks. Further reduction to 5 mg/kg every third day in some cases
- Should be given on an empty stomach to improve absorption of the drug but food may be necessary if vomiting is induced by the drug

Duration
- Usually long term
- Can be used off label with some other drug combinations to reduce dose. Important due to cost issues and reduction of side-effects
  - Glucocorticoids
  - Ketoconazole – no antipruritic effect but may improve cyclosporin utilisation. May reduce cost of cyclosporin in countries where ketoconazole inexpensive
  - Acidic liquids, e.g. grapefruit juice may increase absorption and hence lower dose, but palatability issues render this impractical

Contraindications
- Diabetes mellitus
- Demodicosis
- Dermatophytosis
- Immunosuppressive disease
- Neoplasia
- Deep pyoderma

Adverse effects
- Vomiting, diarrhoea, usually transient
- Gingival hyperplasia
- Very long-term data not yet available as recently licensed

Safety information
- No specific handling instructions for owners
- Gloves should be worn by sensitive individuals

26.4.2 TREATMENT OF SPECIFIC IMMUNE-MEDIATED DISEASES

Pemphigus foliaceus
Principles of treatment
- Can be mild moderate or severe
- Increasingly associated with trigger factors – drugs, infection, food

Primary treatment
- Identify and address possible trigger factors
- Most cases respond to glucocorticoids

- Immunosuppressive doses of prednisolone may be required in the early stages of treatment but maintenance doses are usually low
- Initial dose for 6 weeks then reduce and withdraw to assess resolution
- Maintenance dose for 6 months – if no resolution then repeat reduce and withdraw treatment to assess resolution
- Introduce azathioprine in dogs if non-responsive or dose of prednisolone used leads to unacceptable adverse effects
- Introduce cyclosporin in cats if non-responsive or dose of prednisolone used leads to unacceptable adverse effects
- Introduce cyclosporin in dogs if non-responsive or unacceptable adverse effects with prednisolone and azathioprine

Supportive treatment
- Nutritional support (Chapter 27.4)
- Treat secondary bacterial and yeast infections (Chapter 27.1)

Topical treatment
- Spot treatment with creams and gels may increase patient comfort
- Shampooing will increase patient comfort, remove scale and debris and reduce secondary infection
- Select shampoo according to clinical signs but use the gentlest shampoo indicated
- **See Chapter 29**

Other diseases in the pemphigus complex
- Much less common than pemphigus foliaceus
- Pemphigus vulgaris is usually a more severe disease

Primary treatment
- Mild forms may respond to niacinamide/tetracycline combination therapy
- Most cases require treatment as for pemphigus foliaceus
- Supportive and topical treatment as for pemphigus foliaceus

Bullous pemphigoid
- Rare but usually severe and prognosis guarded

Primary treatment
- Immunosuppressive doses of prednisolone usually required, although maintenance is usually possible on anti-inflammatory doses
- Azathioprine or cyclosporin often required as for pemphigus foliaceus

Supportive and topical treatment as for pemphigus foliaceus
- Shampooing often not indicated due to discomfort caused to patient
- Consider pain relief but do not use non-steroidal anti-inflammatory drugs with glucocorticoids

Adverse cutaneous reactions to drugs
Principles of treatment
- Identify and remove the offending drug
- There is no evidence of a temporal relationship between the use of the drug and the onset of clinical signs

- There is no evidence of a temporal relationship between withdrawal of the drug and the resolution of the clinical signs

Primary treatment
- Usually responsive to glucocorticoids
- Anti-inflammatory doses of glucocorticoids often adequate
- Treat for 6 weeks, then withdraw treatment to assess response

Supportive treatments
- Least is best
- Avoid introduction of other drugs where possible

Topical treatments
- Least is best
- Use warm water showering or mild shampoos to minimise further reactions

Systemic lupus erythematosus
Principles of treatment
- A multisystemic disease complex to diagnose and treat
- Skin signs can be very variable

Primary treatment
- Often responsive to prednisolone, but use with care because of internal organ involvement
- Azathioprine or cyclosporin used in non-responsive cases or where unacceptable adverse effects with prednisolone
- Azathioprine or cyclosporin should be used with care because of internal organ involvement
- Care with azathioprine in cases with blood cell suppression

Supportive treatments
- Skin support should be guided by the need for support for other organs

Topical treatments
- Should be used with care where patient discomfort and systemic illness may be severe
- Pain relief should be considered but systemic illness should influence the choice of drug

Discoid lupus erythematosus
Principles of treatment
- Usually a benign disease which requires only topical treatment
- This is a localised disease which does not usually justify the side-effects associated with systemic treatment
- Often requires long-term control and can be progressive

Primary treatment
- Topical steroid containing creams
- In non-responsive cases anti-inflammatory doses of prednisolone should be used with care

Treatment of Primary Skin Disease

Supportive treatments
- Sunscreens
- Nutritional support may be beneficial

Lupoid onychodystrophy
Principles of treatment
- This can be mild, moderate or severe
- Long-term control is usually required

Primary treatment
- May respond to nutritional support alone
- Some cases respond to niacinamide and tetracycline
- More severe cases require prednisolone
- Azathioprine and cyclosporin should be considered in non-responsive cases and cases where unacceptable adverse effects occur with prednisolone

Supportive treatment
- Nutritional support with vitamin E, zinc and essential fatty acids with cofactors may be beneficial
- Consider pain relief in severe cases and where lameness is present
- Consider protective boots for walks
- Treat secondary bacterial and fungal paronychias
- Keep nails short

Topical treatment
- Always beneficial
- Frequent foot rinsing with warm water
- Antibacterial washes and footbaths

Erythema multiforme
Principles of treatment
- This is a reaction pattern rather than a diagnosis
- The underlying cause should be identified
- Common clinical sign in adverse drug reaction
- Cutaneous adverse reaction to food may result in erythema multiforme

Primary treatment
- In some cases secondary supportive treatments alone are indicated
- Influenced by underlying cause
- Clinical signs usually respond to anti-inflammatory doses of prednisolone
- Azathioprine and cyclosporin may occasionally be indicated

Supportive and topical treatments
- Frequently not indicated

Vasculitis
Principles of treatment
- Many underlying causes

Primary treatment
- Usually responsive to anti-inflammatory doses of glucocorticoids
- Higher doses of glucocorticoids, azathioprine and cyclosporin may be indicated in non-responsive case, or where unacceptable adverse effects occur with prednisolone

26.5   TREATMENT OF ENDOCRINE DISEASE

26.5.1   HYPERADRENOCORTICISM

Pituitary dependent HAC
1   MRI guided laser surgery has been used with some success at one centre
2   Trilostane
3   Mitotane has been used in non-responsive cases under special treatment certificate
4   Others

Adrenal dependent HAC
1   Surgery is treatment of choice where possible but technically demanding
2   Less responsive to trilostane and mitotane therapy than pituitary dependent HAC

Iatrogenic HAC
1   Gradual withdrawal of glucocorticoid treatment
2   The disease which has justified the use of the glucocorticoid treatment may be therapeutically challenging

Ectopic active adrenal tissue
1   Diagnostically challenging
2   Trilostane or mitotane may be used

During the initial treatment intensive supportive treatments may be necessary according to the clinical signs seen (Chapters 27 and 29). It is frequently necessary to continue this support during the course of the treatment although the most severe clinical signs, such as calcinosis cutis, should resolve completely.

Trilostane
Formulation
- Capsules

Mode of action
- Interference with steroid synthesis

Indications
- Pituitary and adrenal dependent HAC

Dose
- An initial dose of 6 mg/kg once daily, adjusted by individual response
- Most dogs are maintained on 2–4 mg/kg daily
- Dosing in the morning facilitates monitoring

Contraindications
- Unconfirmed diagnosis of HAC
- Impaired renal or hepatic function
- Pregnancy or lactation
- Animals intended for breeding

Adverse effects
- May unmask degenerative joint disease and renal disease due to lowering of glucocorticoid levels
- Lethargy, gastrointestinal signs, etc.
- Addisonian crisis
- Sudden death has been reported
- May reduce testosterone synthesis

Safety information
- Women of child bearing age should avoid handling the drug
- May cause hypersensitivity reactions

Monitoring treatment
- Patients should be regularly monitored for side-effects of treatments and destabilisation of the condition by:
  - Regular reassessment of history and clinical signs
  - Water intake where there is polydypsia
  - Blood biochemistry, electrolytes and ACTH stimulation test pre-treatment then at 10 days, 4 weeks, 12 weeks, then every 3 months and after each dose adjustment
  - Samples should be taken 4–6 hours after dose is given
  - Evidence of neurological signs as evidence of tumour spread or metastasis

26.5.2 HYPOTHYROIDISM

Thyroid supplementation is usually necessary.

Increase in dose levels frequently indicated with time due to destruction of supplemented thyroid hormone as well as that produced by patient.

Thyroxine
Formulation
- Oral tablets

Mode of action
- Supplementation of natural thyroxin

Indications
Diagnosed cases of hypothyroidism

Dose
- Commonly used doses of 22 μg/kg are often too low, up to 44 μg/kg are frequently necessary once daily
- Increased dose rates may be required with time due to destruction of exogenous thyroxin

Contraindications
- Thyrotoxicosis
- Adrenal insufficiency
- Care in the presence of cardiovascular disease

Adverse effects
- Prolonged overdosage may result in signs of thyrotoxicosis

Safety information
- Avoid human ingestion

Monitoring treatment
- Side-effects are rare but patients should be regularly monitored
  - Regular reassessment of history and clinical signs
  - Monitor heart rate and rectal temperature
  - Peak and trough free thyroxin levels at intervals before and 4–6 hours after pilling
  - Single sample taken at the same time after pilling on each occasion

During the initial treatment intensive supportive treatments may be necessary according to the clinical signs seen (see Chapters 27 and 29). It is frequently necessary to continue this support during the course of the treatment as clinical signs such as scaling, thinning hair coat and a predilection for secondary pyoderma may remain.

26.5.3   FELINE HYPERTHYROIDISM

The treatment of choice in cases where there is a palpable goitre is surgery following stabilisation of thyroxin levels and clinical signs with carbimazole or methimazole treatment.

Where there is no palpable goitre, radiotherapy should be considered. Cost and radiation safety, along with the effects of stress due to quarantine of the patient are factors in decision making.

Carbimazole or methimazole are frequently used for long-term control of hyperthyroidism, but owners should be warned of the limitations of this option:
- Medical treatment is palliative and does not address the primary tumour
- Blood pressure often stays raised despite reduction in heart rate, so stress on kidneys and heart is not necessarily reduced

Carbimazole
Formulation
- Tablets

Mode of action
- Suppresses thyroxin formation

Indications
- Hyperthyroidism

Dose
- Initially 10–15 mg once daily at the same time of day
- Maintenance usually 10–25 mg once daily
- Other treatments should be used where maintenance is less than 10 mg daily

Treatment of Primary Skin Disease

Contraindications
- Do not use in pregnant or lactating animals
- Avoid in hypersensitive animals
- Thyroid carcinoma

Adverse effects
- Side-effects are not uncommon in doses over 20 mg, so care and careful assessment is needed when using the higher doses
- Raised liver enzymes
- Impaired renal function
- Low red and white blood cell counts
- Thrombocytopaenia

Safety information
- Care with handling; individuals hypersensitive to any of this group of compounds should avoid

Monitoring treatment
- History and clinical signs should be monitored for both side-effects and dose regulation
- Total thyroxin levels should be monitored 10–14 days after a dose change and at 3–6 monthly intervals
- Renal parameters, liver enzymes and complete blood count should be performed at same time as thyroxin levels
- Regular assessment for goitre in the contralateral gland should be performed (70%)

Methimazole/thiamazole
- Oral tablets

Mode of action
- Suppression of thyroxin production

Indications
- Feline hyperthyroidism

Dose
- Initially 2.5 mg twice daily
- Maintenance according to requirements with dosing twice daily where possible
- Care with doses over 10 mg

Contraindications
- Thyroid carcinoma
- Pregnant and lactating animals
- Hypersensitive individuals

Adverse effects
- Hypersensitivity
- Common at doses over 10 mg daily
- Impaired renal function
- Raised liver enzymes
- Suppressed white and red blood cell counts
- Thrombocytopaenia

- 20% of cats
- Facial pruritus

Monitoring treatment
- History and clinical signs should be monitored regularly for both side-effects and dose regulation
- Haematology, biochemistry and serum total thyroxin should be assessed before initiating treatment and after 3 weeks, 6 weeks, 10 weeks, 20 weeks and thereafter every 3 months

26.5.4   DIABETES MELLITUS

Protocols for the primary treatment and control of diabetes mellitus are found in all standard medicine texts and are *not* included in this book.

Secondary dermatological problems should be treated according to the presenting clinical signs (see Chapters 27 and 29).

Where dermatological problems persist a full reassessment of the case should be undertaken as well as ongoing monitoring of blood fructosamine levels.

26.5.5   ADRENAL HYPERPLASIA LIKE SYNDROME (ALOPECIA X, ADRENAL SEX HORMONE IMBALANCE, GROWTH HORMONE RESPONSIVE DERMATOSIS, CASTRATION RESPONSIVE DERMATOSIS)

As this disease frequently only causes cosmetic issues, the owner may not elect to treat the condition.

Melatonin has been used with success at doses of 3–6 mg twice daily. There is no change in sex hormones but hair regrowth is seen. This is available online as a food supplement.

Mitotane and trilostane have also been used but it is controversial as to whether a drug which is used off label and has the potential for serious side-effects should be used. Various other sex hormone therapies have been used in small numbers of cases.

Secondary dermatological problems should be treated according to the presenting clinical signs (see Chapters 27 and 29).

Monitoring treatment
- The patient should be assessed at regular intervals for side-effects of treatment and progression or development of systemic signs which may be suggestive of hyperadrenocorticism
- Improved hair growth may be temporary

26.5.6   TESTICULAR OR OVARIAN TUMOURS OR DYSFUNCTION

The treatment of choice for these problems is removal of the gonads.

Secondary dermatological problems should resolve following treatment of the primary problem but should be treated according to the presenting clinical signs (see Chapters 27 and 29).

Treatment of Primary Skin Disease

26.5.7   PITUITARY DWARFISM

Some patients are euthanased due to behavioural problems.

No primary treatment is available.

Dermatological signs are usually controlled by addressing the presenting clinical signs (see Chapters 27 and 29).

26.6   TREATMENTS FOR HAIR FOLLICLE DISORDERS AND KERATINISATION DEFECTS (PRIMARY SCALING DISORDERS, PRIMARY SEBORRHOEA)

26.6.1   PRIMARY TREATMENTS USED

The list of primary treatments commonly used in primary scaling disorders is listed in Table 26.10.

Vitamin A
Formulation
• Capsules

Mode of action
• Supplementation

Indications for use
• Vitamin A responsive dermatosis

Dose
• 10,000 IU once daily with a fatty meal lifelong

Contraindications
• Care in pregnancy

Table 26.10   Specific treatments for some primary scaling conditions

Condition	Treatments
Vitamin A and zinc responsive dermatoses	High level supplementation and dietary correction where necessary
Sebaceous adenitis	Synthetic retinoids, cyclosporin, glucocorticoids, essential fatty acids
Ichthyosis	Synthetic retinoids
Idiopathic facial dermatitis	Palliative only
Hair follicle dysplasias	Palliative only
Nasodigital hyperplasias, ear margin dermatosis	Palliative only
Schnauzer comedo syndrome	Palliative only
Lichenoid psoriasiform dermatosis	Palliative only
Primary keratinisation defect	Palliative only

Please note that some of the drugs used here do not have a veterinary licence and those licensed are being used in a manner other than their data sheet recommendations. They should only be used with the fully informed consent of the owners.

Adverse effects
- None except in overdose

Safety information
- Normal handling precautions

Zinc sulphate
- Formulation
- 200 mg capsules

Mode of action
- Supplementation

Indications for use
- Zinc responsive dermatosis
- Zinc may be added to diets as a supplement for inflamed skin

Dose
- 200 mg daily for zinc responsive dermatosis for 6 weeks
- Less for anti-inflammatory supplementation

Contraindications
- None reported

Adverse effects
- Toxic in overdose
- Can be gastric irritant. Can be addressed by opening capsules and sprinkling contents over food

Safety information
- None

Isotretinoin
- The use of this drug in animal patients is off label. Written informed consent should be obtained from owners to ensure they understand the potential for side-effects and safety information.

Formulation
- Capsules 5 mg and 20 mg

Mode of action
- Synthetic retinoid, mimicking actions of high dose vitamin A with less toxicity

Indications for use
- Sebaceous adenitis
- Other primary keratinisation defects

Dose
- 1–3 mg/kg daily for 3 months initially
- Withdraw treatment to assess response
- Can be kept on treatment long term

Contraindications
- Pregnancy and lactation
- Should not be used in animals intended for breeding
- Liver or kidney disease

Adverse effects
- Raised liver enzymes
- Hepatopathy
- Very teratogenic
- Depression in humans
- Dry eye

Safety information
- Should not be handled by women of child bearing age
- Gloves should be worn to handle the product

Prednisolone
Formulation
- Oral tablets

Mode of action
- Gene repression of multiple transcription factors for cytokines and their receptors, chemotactic proteins, adhesion molecules and pro-inflammatory enzymes
- Prevents the activation of many immune cells, e.g. T cells, eosinophils, macrophages and dendritic cells
- Can also activate anti-inflammatory genes

Indications
- Moderate to severe cases of immune-mediated disease as first line treatment
- Non-responsive cases of mild to moderate immune-mediated disease

Dose
- Mild to moderate disease – dogs 1–2 mg/kg; cats 1–3 mg/kg
- Moderate to severe disease – immunosuppressive doses – dogs 2–4 mg/kg; cats 3–6 mg/kg
- Where a trigger factor can be identified and addressed short courses of 6 weeks may be sufficient
- Where a trigger factor cannot be identified, treatment should be withdrawn gradually after 6 weeks and again after 6 months to 'test' for resolution
- After initial treatment for 6 weeks, alternate day dosing should be initiated and the lowest possible maintenance dose achieved (see Chapter 28)

Contraindications
- Diabetes mellitus
- Demodicosis
- Dermatophytosis
- Immunosuppressive disease
- Neoplasia
- Infectious disease

Adverse effects
- As these are dose dependent, they are more common and more severe at immunosuppressive doses
- Polydypsia/polyuria
- Polyphagia and scavenging
- Muscle, tendon and ligament weakening
- Hyperadrenocorticism

- Diabetes mellitus
- Pancreatitis
- Hepatolipidosis
- Secondary urinary tract infections

Safety information
- Some patients may be depressed or show changes in behaviour on glucocorticoids

Cyclosporin
Formulation
- Capsules

Indications for use
- Off label use for moderate to severe immune-mediated disease
- May be used off label concomitantly with prednisolone to reduce the dose of steroid required

Mode of action
- T cell activation inhibitor
- T cell cytokine inhibitor
- Mast cell inhibitor
- Reduced eosinophil survival

Dose
- Initial dose of 5 mg/kg daily, reducing to 5 mg/kg every other day after 6 weeks. Further reduction to 5 mg/kg every third day in some cases
- Should be given on an empty stomach to improve absorption of the drug, but food may be necessary if vomiting is induced by the drug

Duration
- Usually long term
- Can be used off label with some other drug combinations to reduce dose. Important due to cost issues and reduction of side-effects
- Glucocorticoids
- Ketoconazole – no antipruritic effect but may improve cyclosporin utilisation
- May reduce cost of cyclosporin in countries where ketoconazole inexpensive
- Acidic liquids, e.g. grapefruit juice may increase absorption and hence lower dose, but palatability issues render this impractical

Contraindications
- Diabetes mellitus
- Demodicosis
- Dermatophytosis
- Immunosuppressive disease
- Neoplasia
- Deep pyoderma

Adverse effects
- Vomiting, diarrhoea, usually transient
- Gingival hyperplasia
- Very long-term data not yet available as recently licensed

Safety information
- No specific handling instructions for owners
- Gloves should be worn by sensitive individuals

26.6.2 TREATMENT OF DISEASES CAUSING KERATINISATION DEFECTS

Vitamin A responsive dermatosis
Principles of treatment
- Long-term control is usually necessary

Primary treatment
- Vitamin A supplementation

Supportive treatment
- Treat secondary bacterial and yeast infections
- Ear canals may need special attention due to accumulation of scale and debris

Topical treatments
- Shampooing is always beneficial
- The mildest keratolytic keratoplastic shampoos should be used where possible
- See Chapter 29

Zinc responsive dermatosis
Principles of treatment
- Correct possibly zinc deficient diets
- Zinc enriched diets
- Zinc supplementation

Primary treatment
- 200 mg zinc sulphate daily in food for 6 weeks, while diet is addressed

Supportive treatment
- Treat secondary bacterial and yeast infections

Topical treatments
- Shampooing is always beneficial
- The mildest keratolytic keratoplastic shampoos should be used where possible
- See Chapter 29

Sebaceous adenitis
Principles of treatment
- Rapid treatment to prevent loss of further pilosebaceous units, which is permanent
- Anti-inflammatory treatment for increased patient comfort

Primary treatment
- Isotretinoin is the most frequently prescribed drug, but this is an off label use of this drug and great care should be taken in detailing the adverse effects and safety information. Written consent should be obtained.

Supplementary treatment
- Treat secondary bacterial and yeast infections (see Chapters 27 and 29)
- Treat scaling symptomatically (see Chapters 27 and 29)

Topical treatment
- Shampooing is always beneficial to improve scaling (see Chapter 29)
- Protection from sunburn may be necessary when dorsal hairloss is extensive
- Protection from cold may be necessary when dorsal hairloss is extensive

Ichthyosis
Principles of treatment
- Mild cases may not require treatment
- Topical treatments may be sufficient in mild to moderate disease to control scaling

Primary treatment
- Isotretinoin is occasionally used, but this is an off label use of this drug and great care should be taken in detailing the adverse effects and safety information. Written consent should be obtained.

Supplementary treatment
- Treat secondary bacterial and yeast infections (see Chapters 27 and 29)
- Treat scaling symptomatically (see Chapters 27 and 29)

Topical treatment
- Shampooing is always beneficial to improve scaling (see Chapter 29)

Other hair follicle disorders
Secondary hair follicle disorders are common and the underlying cause should be addressed.

Primary hair follicle disorders are rare and are often either genetic or congenital. Apart from sebaceous adenitis most hair follicle disorders can only be treated by palliation, according to the presenting clinical signs (see Chapters 27 and 29).

26.7 CHEMOTHERAPEUTIC AGENTS COMMONLY USED IN SKIN NEOPLASIA

This section is largely to make the practitioner familiar with the drugs which might be used for chemotherapy of skin cancer patients.

All of these are used off label (with the exception of prednisolone and cyclosporin) and do not have a veterinary licence.

All of these drugs (with the exception of water) have the potential for serious adverse effects.

Current protocols should be sought before treating any patient with these drugs and the data sheet for each product read carefully. Those with limited expertise or facilities for the use of these drugs should consider referral to an oncologist.

Treatment of Primary Skin Disease

The owner should be given full details of the potential for adverse effect and written informed consent should be received.

Local regulations should be followed regarding the disposal of all material used with these agents.

There are serious health and safety implications for the staff and owners handling these patients and their waste. Adequate precautions should be taken.

Lomustine
(1-[2-chlorethyl] 3-cyclohexyl-1-nitrosurea, CCNU)

Formulation
- Capsules

Mode of action
- Non-specific alkylating agent
- Binds to DNA strands, inserts alkyl, inhibits protein synthesis

Indications
- All off label use
- Mainly anecdotal and small number case reports
- Lymphoma, including epitheliotrophic lymphoma and mast cell tumour
- Series of epitheliotrophic lymphoma treated with lomustine with success and acceptable side-effects

Dose
- Dose rates of 60–90 mg/m² have been reported, but standard texts should be referred to for most recent protocols

Adverse effects
- Gastrointestinal effects most common
- Anaemia and thrombocytopaenia
- Lethargy
- Hepatopathy
- Other
- Reduced resistance to infection

Vincrystine

Formulation
- Dry powder for reconstitution using fume cupboard or device for reducing aerosol formation and intravenous injection
- Perivascular injection is extremely irritant and likely to result in tissue sloughs

Mode of action
- Inhibits mitosis

Indications
- Multicentric lymphoma, mast cell tumours, epitheliotrophic lymphoma

Adverse effects
- Gastrointestinal effects
- Peripheral neuropathy
- Lowered resistance to infection

Doxorubicin
Formulation
- Red fluid for intravenous injection
- Perivascular injection is extremely irritant and likely to result in tissue sloughs

Mode of action
- Binds to and breaks DNA strands
- Binding to cell membranes and altering ion transport
- Generation of oxygen radicals

Indications
- Conditions non-responsive to other chemotherapy protocols

Adverse effects
- Gastrointestinal effects the most common
- Heart arrhythmias
- Reduced resistance to infection

Methotrexate
Formulation
- Tablets
- Or yellow fluid for intravenous injection
- Perivascular injection is very irritant

Mode of action
- Inhibits folic acid metabolism

Indications
- Occasionally used as part of a multidrug combination in lymphoma

Adverse effects
- Bone marrow suppression
- Gastrointestinal disorders
- Anaemia

Cyclophosphamide
Formulation
- Tablets or liquid for intravenous injection

Mode of action
- Alkylating agent

Adverse effects
- Gastrointestinal disorders
- Bone marrow suppression
- Anaemia
- Hepatopathy

Chlorambucil
Formulation
- Tablets

Mode of action
- Alkylating agent

Adverse effects
- Bone marrow suppression
- Loss of appetite and gastrointestinal upsets
- Anaemia

Masitinib mesylate
- Licensed for the treatment of mast cell tumours in dogs where tumours are unresectable and the presence of a mutated tyrosine kinase c-kit receptor has been confirmed

Formulation
- Tablets

Mode of action
- Protein-tyrosine kinase inhibitor

Adverse effects
- Most common are mild to moderate gastrointestinal side-effects
- Contraindicated in some liver and kidney problems, anaemia and neutropaenia
- Should not be used in animals less than 4 kg or less than 6 months of age

Water
- Intralesional injection of water has been advocated for the treatment of mast cell tumours but a recent study does not support its use

Prednisolone and cyclosporin
- Prednisolone and cyclosporin are frequently used for their anti-inflammatory effect and as palliation

Chapter 27

Treatment of Presenting Signs

27.1 MANAGEMENT OF PRURITUS

Pruritic skin disease is distressing and frustrating for client, patient and veterinarian.

It has been said that inflammatory skin disease accounts for about 25% of veterinary visits of sick pets and that about 15% of the canine population suffers from hypersensitivity dermatitis.

27.1.1 ACUTE SHORT DURATION/NON-RECURRENT EPISODES OF PRURITUS

Acute short duration/non-recurrent episodes of pruritus can be treated without investigation of the underlying cause.

- Localised dermatitis where the possibility of demodicosis or dermatophytosis has been excluded
- Hives and urticaria which are non-recurrent and short-lived
- Single occurrence of acute moist dermatitis where anal sac or flea related disease have been excluded
- Generalised dermatitis where the underlying cause can reasonably be considered to have been removed (e.g. contact irritants) or of short duration (e.g. seasonal atopic dermatitis)

27.1.2 WHERE IT IS NOT POSSIBLE TO IDENTIFY AND ADDRESS THE UNDERLYING CAUSE

Where it is not possible to identify and address the underlying cause symptomatic treatment of pruritus is justified for patient comfort.

Reasons include:
- Owner compliance for diagnostic tests
- Underlying cause remains obscure despite diagnostic investigation
- Treatment of underlying cause not available
- Treatment of underlying cause non-responsive or only partially responsive to treatment

Even in these cases, however, it is important to exclude the presence of dermatophytosis, demodicosis, microbial disease and immunosuppressive or systemic disease before the use of symptomatic treatment.

27.1.3 SYMPTOMATIC CONTROL OF PRURITUS IS OFTEN NECESSARY AS AN ADJUNCTIVE TREATMENT

Symptomatic control of pruritus is often necessary as an adjunctive treatment during the treatment of some diagnosed conditions:

- Scabies
- Flea bite dermatitis
- Otacariasis
- Severe cheyletiellosis and louse infestation
- Harvest mite dermatitis
- Hypersensitivity dermatitis
- Acute moist dermatitis
- *Malassezia* dermatitis

27.1.4 THE INVESTIGATION OF PRURITIC SKIN DISEASE

The investigation of pruritic skin disease is described in Chapter 4.

To summarise persistent or recurrent pruritic skin disease should always be investigated as follows:

- History and full clinical examination
- Dermatological examination
- Examination for and treatment of ectoparasitic problems
- Investigation of the possibility of dermatophytosis
- Investigation of the possibility of other infectious disease
- Evidence of concurrent systemic disease
- Evidence of concurrent immunosuppressive disease

27.1.5 CONTROL OF PRURITUS

Control of pruritus should be considered very carefully in the following conditions where the use of some antipruritic drugs is contraindicated:

- Demodicosis
- Dermatophytosis
- Pyoderma
- Concurrent infectious disease
- Hyperadrenocorticism
- Diabetes mellitus
- Other systemic disease
- Immunosuppressive disease

27.1.6 CONSTANT REVIEW

Constant review of the pruritic condition is required.

Treatment of Presenting Signs

Review of underlying diagnosis
- Addition of new allergens in atopic dermatitis, e.g. seasonal, food
- Concomitant disease
- Misdiagnosis should be considered and diagnosis reviewed

Flare factors exacerbate pruritus
- Concomitant flea bite dermatitis
- Change in environmental conditions, e.g. heat and humidity
- Seasonal hypersensitivities
- Secondary infections

Concomitant disease
- Atopic dogs are more likely to suffer from flea bite dermatitis
- New hypersensitivities may develop
- Other pruritic disease may develop

Complications of treatment
- Increased risk of microbial infection and drug induced skin reactions
- Diabetes mellitus and hyperadrenocorticism with glucocorticoids
- Dry hair coat, hairloss and scaling with glucocorticoids
- Demodicosis with immunosuppressive drugs
- Progression of pyoderma (Chapter 27.2)

Inflammatory diseases progress with time
- Primary disease becomes refractory to treatment
- Chronic changes in skin less amenable to treatment
- Chronic changes in skin predispose to flare factors and secondary complications
- Superantigens in staphylococci infections
- Self-perpetuating inflammation in hypersensitivity dermatitis
- Chronic inflammatory change exacerbates the primary defect in inflammatory disease

27.1.7 METHODS OF CONTROLLING PRURITUS

Primary treatment of the primary disease
- Avoidance of cause
- Immunomodulation (generally only available for atopic dermatitis)
- Drug therapy
- For detailed description see Chapter 4, Section 3 and Chapter 26.

Primary effect on pruritus using drugs
- Drugs to control inflammation or itch, e.g. glucocorticoids, cyclosporin and antihistamines

Prevent further damage to the epidermal barrier
- Prevent further damage by control of pruritus
- Supplement the epidermal barrier with essential fatty acid and cofactor containing supplements and foods

- Essential fatty acid containing shampoos
- Address the primary disease

Control secondary effects on coat condition and scaling
- See Chapters 27 and 29
- Essential fatty acids
- Chinese herbal supplements
- Nutritional support (Chapter 27.4)
- Shampoos and topical treatments (Chapter 29)

Treatment and control of flare factors
- Topical and systemic antibacterial treatments (Chapters 27.2, 29)
- Topical and systemic anti-yeast treatments (Chapters 27.2, 29)
- Removal of irritant products of inflammation (Chapter 29)
- Removal of scale, bacteria and yeasts from skin (Chapters 27.3, 29)

Emollients and other soothing treatments
See Chapter 29
- Frequent warm water showering or bathing
- Antipruritic shampoos
- Moisturising shampoos
- Keratoplastic and keratolytic shampoos
- Antimicrobial shampoos

27.1.8 TREATMENTS AVAILABLE FOR THE CONTROL OF PRURITUS

There are many drugs available for the control of pruritus. As treatment is likely to be long term, the following factors are important:

- Evidence for efficacy
- Side-effects, both in short- and long-term use
- Contraindications
- Label restrictions
- Ease of administration
- Drug interactions
- Cost

Glucocorticoids
Remain the mainstay for pruritus control in the dog and cat. Also used off label in the other small mammals.

Formulations
- Oral tablets
- Creams, gels ointments
- Sprays

Mode of action
- Gene repression of multiple transcription factors for cytokines and their receptors, chemotactic proteins, adhesion molecules and pro-inflammatory enzymes
- Prevents the activation of many immune cells, e.g. T cells, eosinophils, macrophages and dendritic cells
- Can also activate anti-inflammatory genes

Short-term use of glucocorticoids
Indications
- Supportive treatment of ectoparasitic disease (except demodicosis)
- Acute moist dermatitis
- Hives, urticaria, cutaneous anaphylaxis
- Short-term treatment of flare factors
- Insect bites stings
- Seasonal atopic dermatitis
- Acute onset single incident pruritic skin disease

Dose
- 1–2 mg/kg prednisolone or methylprednisolone daily initially for 14 days. If longer-term use is required taper dose to maintenance dose of 0.5 mg/kg daily after 10–14 days
- Short-term dosing of glucocorticoids should be used only for a maximum of 6 weeks on a single occasion. If further use of glucocorticoids is considered the diagnosis should be reviewed (see Chapter 4)

Longer-term use of glucocorticoids
Indications
- Only oral prednisolone and methylprednisolone are suitable for the long-term control of pruritus
- Until recently there were few published trials on the efficacy of glucocorticoids, but several clinical trials for other drugs have used glucocorticoids as 'gold standard', so more information is available now
- Diagnosed cases of pruritic skin disease only
- Hypersensitivity dermatitis and immune-mediated disease

Duration
- Long-term dosing of glucocorticoids is often necessary
- There is no safe minimum dose of glucocorticoids, but all efforts should be made to reduce the dose used
- There is evidence that alternate day dosing is safer than daily dosing even when the same total dose is used
- Slow tapering (reduce dose by 50% every 3 weeks) usually allows a lower maintenance dose to be achieved
- Long-term low dose maintenance generally gives better control and fewer side-effects than repeated short courses of higher dose treatment where glucocorticoid treatment is necessary for more than 50% of the time
- Where long-term use of glucocorticoids is necessary, steroid sparing measures should always be considered

Steroid sparing measures
- Treat flare factors
  - Secondary infection
  - Concurrent ectoparasitic disease
  - Removal of irritant skin debris
- Topical treatments (see Chapter 29)
- Drug combinations. Concurrent use of a number of other drugs allows a reduction in the dose of glucocorticoids. Nearly all of these combinations involve the off label use of one, some or all of the drugs used
  - Cyclosporin
  - Antihistamines
  - Essential fatty acid supplementation
  - Chinese herbal supplementation

Contraindications for the use of glucocorticoids
- Demodicosis
- Dermatophytosis
- Other infectious disease
- Concurrent systemic disease, especially
  - Diabetes mellitus
  - Hyperadrenocorticism
  - Liver disease
  - Bacterial, viral or fungal disease
  - Immunosuppressive disease
- Where any of the above is suspected and not ruled out

Adverse effects
- Polydypsia/polyuria
- Polyphagia and scavenging
- Muscle, tendon and ligament weakening
- Hyperadrenocorticism
- Diabetes mellitus
- Pancreatitis
- Hepatolipidosis
- Secondary urinary tract infections

Safety information
- Gloves should be worn for the administration of all topical preparations
- Sprays should be used in a well ventilated area
- Avoid the treatment of large areas of skin with topical treatments
- Steroids should only be used long term where a diagnosis of chronic responsive disease such as hypersensitivity dermatitis or immune-mediated disease has been made
- Steroid sparing measures should be introduced when long-term use is considered

Cyclosporin
Formulation
- Capsules

Indications for use
- Atopic dermatitis

Mode of action
- T cell activation inhibitor
- T cell cytokine inhibitor
- Mast cell inhibitor
- Reduced eosinophil survival

Dose
- Initial dose 5 mg/kg daily without food
- In most cases a dose reduction to 5 mg/kg every other day can be made after 6 weeks
- In some cases a further dose reduction to 5 mg/kg every third day can be made after a further 6 weeks
- Should be given on an empty stomach to improve absorption of the drug, but food may be necessary if vomiting is induced by the drug
- Licensed for the treatment of atopic dermatitis in dogs

Duration
- Usually long term
- Can be used off label with some other drug combinations to reduce dose. Important due to cost issues and reduction of side-effects
- Glucocorticoids
- Ketoconazole – no antipruritic effect but may improve cyclosporin utilisation
- May reduce cost of cyclosporin in countries where ketoconazole inexpensive
- Acidic liquids, e.g. grapefruit juice may increase absorption and hence lower the dose required, but palatability issues

Contraindications
- Neoplasia
- Deep pyoderma
- Diabetes mellitus, but can be used with caution and reference to manufacturer

Adverse effects
- Vomiting, diarrhoea, usually transient, occasionally persistent colic
- Hirsuitism
- Gingival hyperplasia
- May be associated with T cell depression in long-term use

Safety information
- No particular handling restrictions for humans
- Should be withdrawn before vaccination or dead vaccines considered

Antihistamines
- There is conflicting evidence for the efficacy of many of the antihistamines
- There are no antihistamines licensed for use in small animals. These drugs are used off label and some of the drugs may show undesirable side-effects
- Many human antihistamine drugs have been used in the control of atopic dermatitis
- There is some evidence to support efficacy for a combination of hydroxyzine and chlorpheniramine
- Antihistamines may also be useful in reducing the dose of glucocorticoids necessary to control pruritus

Mode of action
- Act via H1 receptionists against the effects of histamine release
- May also alter lymphocyte proliferative responses, chemotaxis and antibody synthesis

Dose
- 7–14 day trials should be carried out of each antihistamine to determine if any are effective
- An improvement of between 10% and 30% has been reported in some individuals using some of the drugs
- These drugs are not licensed for use in dogs and cats, so dose rates are largely anecdotal and there have been few controlled trials of their use
- See Table 27.1

Indications
- Mild to moderate pruritus where the underlying cause is known to be transient (e.g. insect bite or sting) or where the underlying cause has been addressed
- May be effective in mild atopic dermatitis where there is minimal secondary change

Contraindications
- Should not be used where a veterinary licensed product can be used safely and effectively
- Should not be used in pregnant or young animals

Adverse effects
- May cause drowsiness
- Beware of drug combinations as unexpected side-effects are possible
- Terfinadine and asemizole should be avoided as they may cause cardiac arrhythmias in the dog

Safety information
- Generally safe, but antihistamines have been measured in milk of lactating patients, so human care with handling

Essential fatty acids
- These have been used in high doses in recent years, following work on their effectiveness in reducing pruritus
- There have been insufficient adequately controlled studies to demonstrate efficacy in reducing pruritus

Table 27.1 Some suggested dose rates of antihistamines which have been shown to have some beneficial effect

Generic name	Dog dose	Cat dose
Chlorpheniramine	Up to 0.4 mg/kg bid/tid	2 mg bid
Diphenhydramine	2 mg/kg bid/tid	2 mg/kg bid/tid
Hydroxyzine	2–3 mg/kg bid/tid	10 mg bid/tid
Clemastine	0.05–1 mg/kg bid	No data
Loratidine	5–20 mg/kg sid/bid	5 mg sid/bid
Cetrizine	5–20 mg/kg bid	5 mg sid/bid

- Essential fatty acid supplementation is however beneficial in pruritic patients to improve coat condition and scaling and also to aid tissue repair in skin damage

Proposed modes of action
- Modulate prostaglandin synthesis to favour anti-inflammatory metabolites
- Suppress leukotriene synthesis
- Inhibit cell activation and cytokine secretion
- Correct epidermal lipid defects

Contraindications
- Intolerance to ingredients

Adverse effects
- Rare, may cause loose stools

Safety information
- None

Chinese herbal supplement
- Recently introduced based on a human Chinese traditional remedy, but with fewer herbs. There is some evidence that this may be a useful adjunct in the control of pruritus due to atopic dermatitis

Kinase inhibitors
A number of kinase inhibitors are under investigation for use in atopic dermatitis.

Other drugs which have been used off label for the control of pruritus.

Although licensed for use in humans the safety and efficacy of these drugs has not been tested in dogs and cats, therefore their use should be reserved for a last resort, and clients should be warned before use. Dose rates and frequencies have not been fully evaluated in our species.

- Misoprostol, some benefit reported
- Tacrolimus ointment, some benefit reported, inadvisable due to reported hazards of human handling
- Pentoxyfylline has shown some benefit with a low incidence of side-effects
- Leukotriene inhibitors, no evidence for beneficial effect in dogs and cats
- Fluoxetine has been used with some success in the treatment of acral lick of dermatitis, but there is no evidence for a beneficial effect in treatment of pruritus in dogs and cats
- Topical capsaicin, insufficient evidence for beneficial effect in pruritus

27.2 BACTERIAL AND YEAST INFECTIONS

27.2.1 BACTERIAL PYODERMA

Pyoderma is important in skin disease but is usually secondary to an underlying cause (Chapters 7 and 11).

Principles of treatment of pyoderma
1 Address the underlying cause
2 Use an appropriate antibacterial agent
3 Use the correct dose for the patient
4 Use the correct dose for an adequate period of time
5 Use suitable adjunctive and supportive treatments
6 Review underlying cause, treatment plan and client compliance at regular intervals
7 Avoid the use of potentially immunosuppressive anti-inflammatory drugs during treatment

Address the underlying cause of the pyoderma
'Healthy adult skin does not normally become infected.'

Primary pyoderma is rare. Except where the condition is mild and transient the underlying cause should be determined for effective treatment.

The common underlying causes of pyoderma are described in the following sections.

- Ectoparasites (Chapter 10)
- Micro-organisms (Chapter 11)
- Hypersensitivity dermatitis (Chapter 12)
- Immune-mediated disease (Chapter 13)
- Endocrine skin disease (Chapter 14)
- Hair follicle disorders (Chapter 15)
- Neoplasia (Chapter 16)
- Other skin disease (Chapter 17)

Pyoderma is a common secondary complicating or flare factor in many dermatoses.

Problem oriented approach to skin disease (Section 2) should be used to identify the underlying cause and treat it. Where the underlying cause is well controlled, there may be little or no need for treatment of pyoderma.

Pyoderma should always be considered and treated when a flare of clinical signs is suspected.

Pyoderma, if mistreated may progress to a deeper, more refractory form (Figure 27.1).

Use an appropriate antibacterial agent
In general it is more important how an antibacterial agent is used rather than which one is chosen.

In chronic or recurrent cases bacterial culture, identification and sensitivity should be undertaken from the contents of an intact pustule (culture of ruptured lesions or surface is useless as contaminant, commensal and transient organisms will be cultured).

In mild or transient pyoderma topical treatments alone may be sufficient (see Chapter 29), but in most cases of superficial or deep pyoderma a systemic antibiotic is necessary.

A list of antibacterial agents frequently used in the treatment of pyoderma is shown in Table 27.2.

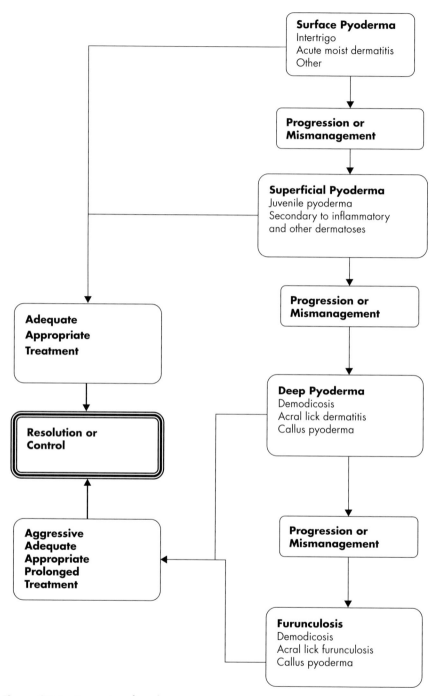

Figure 27.1   Progression of pyoderma.

Table 27.2 Systemic antibiotics useful in the treatment of pyoderma

Group	Generic name	Formulation	Dose/kg	Duration
Cephalosporins (bactericidal, inhibit bacterial cell wall synthesis)	Cephalexin	Tablet/oral drops	15 mg/kg twice daily	5–28 days, longer at clinician's discretion depending on brand
	Cefovecin	Injection	8 mg/kg	Every 14 days × 4
Potentiated penicillins (inhibit cell wall synthesis and an enzyme)	Clavulanic acid potentiated amoxicillin	Tablet	12.5 mg/kg twice daily	5–20 days, longer at clinician's discretion, depending on brand
Fluoroquinolones (interfere with DNA synthesis)	Orbifloxacin	Tablets	7.5 mg/kg once daily	Not stated
	Enrofloxacin	Tablets	5 mg/kg once daily	3–10 days, do not exceed dose or duration in cats
	Enrofloxacin	Liquid	Small mammals 5 mg/kg twice daily Reptiles 5 mg/kg once daily Birds 10 mg/kg twice daily	7 days 6 days 7 days
	Marbofloxacin	Tablets	2 mg/kg once daily	Up to 28 days in dogs, 3–5 days in cats
	Ibafloxin	Gel	15 mg/kg once daily	10 days, 21 days for deep pyoderma
Lincosides (interfere with protein synthesis)	Clindamycin	Capsules	11 mg/kg either once daily or in divided doses	7–10 days, up to maximum of 28 days on clinical judgement, depending on brand
	Lincomycin	Tablets	22 mg/kg twice daily	Not stated
Potentiated sulphonamides (interfere with DNA synthesis and inhibit an enzyme)	Trimethoprim/ sulphadiazine		30 mg/kg once daily or in divided doses	Up to 5 days or until 2 days after resolution
Tetracyclins (interfere with protein synthesis)	Doxycline (tetracyclin)	Tablets	Dogs and cats 10 mg/kg once daily Pigeons and cagebirds 15mg/ kg once daily	Up to 5 days (treatment of pyoderma off label use) 5 days or longer (treatment of skin infections is off label use)

Treatment of Presenting Signs

Table 27.3 shows some antibacterial agents which have occasionally been used in the treatment of canine and feline pyoderma following bacterial culture and sensitivity results. **The diagnosis of underlying disease should be reconsidered before using these drugs.**

Table 27.4 lists the antibacterial agents commonly found in topical treatments.

In making a choice of antibiotic many factors should be taken into consideration.

- Fluoroquinolones should be avoided in young animals
- Long courses of fluoroquinolones should be avoided, especially in cats
- The potential of adverse reactions such as hypersensitivity and nephrotoxicity
- Ease of delivery
    - Owner compliance may be greater with less frequent dosing
    - Ease of administration of oral drops, tablets and capsules vary
    - Injectables may be considered if owner/patient compliance is unlikely

Special consideration should be given to the possible adverse effects of off label use of these drugs for longer courses often indicated for superficial and deep pyoderma.

There is a limited choice of suitable veterinary licensed products for the treatment of skin infections in the minor species.

When choosing a second antibiotic in non-responsive pyoderma,
1   Reconsider and readdress the underlying cause
2   Bacterial culture and sensitivity is mandatory
3   Choose an antibiotic from a different functional group
4   Consider cross reactions for bacterial resistance between lincosides and macrolides

In mild or transient cases, or in cases of surface pyoderma, topical treatments alone may be effective. Topical treatments have limitations when used on their own (Chapter 29) but can often be effective in localised lesions and a useful adjunct to treatment of generalised dermatoses.

Sprays and powders licensed for other species should be avoided.

Older formulations, such as powders and cleansing solutions, should be used with care to avoid irritant reactions.

Use the correct dose
The dose rates for the commonly used systemic antibacterial agents are given in Table 27.2.

- The dose rate of the drug to be given should be known
- The patient should be weighed to allow the correct dose to be calculated accurately
- Consult the data sheet for factors which may affect blood levels, such as feeding, concurrent drug use, health, maturity and weight status
- It is tempting to opt for a lower dose when using expensive antibiotics, but this is false economy and ineffective
- The use of a double dose of some antibiotics in superficial and deep pyoderma has been advocated, but there is little evidence to back this up in most cases
- Low dose long-term therapy has been advocated in chronic or recurrent pyoderma, but there is little evidence to support this. This use is controversial and may favour resistance

Table 27.3 Some antibiotics which have occasionally been used off label in pyoderma

Cefadroxil *Cephalosporin*	2 mg/kg twice daily
Oxacillin *Penicillin*	2 mg/kg 3 times daily
Erythromcycin *Macrolide*	15 mg/kg 3 times daily
Clarythromycin *Macrolide*	5–10 mg/kg twice daily
Difloxacin *Fluoroquinolone*	5–10 mg/kg twice daily
Ormetoprim/sulfadimethoxine *Potentiated sulphonamide*	55 mg/kg once daily
Bacquiloprim/sulfadimethoxine *Potentiated sulphonamide*	30 mg/kg Daily for 2 days then alternative days
Tylosin *Macrolide*	10–20 mg/kg twice daily
Doxycline *Tetracyclin*	10 mg/kg once daily for up to 5 days
Rifampicin *Rifamycin*	5–10 mg/kg once daily

These agents are used off licence and dose rates are a guide only.
They should not be used empirically, only following supportive culture and sensitivity results.

Table 27.4 Antibacterial agents frequently used in topical treatments

Active ingredient	Formulation	Indications	Frequency of use	Duration of use
Benzoyl peroxide	Shampoo	Pyoderma	Daily to monthly	As needed
Selenium sulphide	Shampoo	Pyoderma	Weekly	As needed
Chlorhexidine	Shampoo	Pyoderma	Twice weekly	As needed
Chlortetracyclin	Powder	Wounds	Once daily or more	As needed
Fusidic acid	Gel	Surface pyoderma	Twice daily	5–7 days
Neomycin/thiostrepton	Ointment	Localised pyoderma	Up to 3 times daily	As needed
Mupiricin (off label)	Cream	Pyoderma where steroids contraindicated	Three times daily	10 days
Polymixin B	Suspension	Pyoderma	Twice daily	2–3 weeks
Propylene glycol, malic, benzoic and salicylic acids	Cream or solution	Necrotic infected wounds	Dependent on the product containing the active ingredient	Dependent on the product containing the active ingredient

- Pulse dosing of antibiotics (e.g. 1 week off, then 1 week on repeated) has been advocated in chronic or recurrent pyoderma, but there is little evidence to support this. This use is controversial and may favour resistance

Use the antibacterial drug for long enough

Surface pyoderma
- Systemic antibiotics frequently unnecessary, where used a course of 5–7 days is usually sufficient
- Topical treatments should be used beyond clinical cure

Superficial pyoderma
- In mild or localised superficial pyoderma topical treatments alone may be sufficient, used beyond clinical cure
- In transient cases 10–14 days of systemic antibiotics are usually sufficient
- In chronic or recurrent pyoderma a course of 3–6 weeks minimum is required. Systemic antibiotics should be continued for 2 weeks beyond clinical cure

Deep pyoderma
- A minimum of 6 weeks systemic antibiotics should be given, at least 3 weeks beyond clinical cure
- In many cases courses of 6 months or more may be necessary and in some cases permanent control of pyoderma is necessary

Furunculosis
- Systemic antibiotic treatment is usually necessary for several months, as the embedded keratin provides a nidus for bacterial infection. In some cases, permanent control of pyoderma is necessary

Use suitable adjunctive and supportive treatments
- The use of adjunctive and supportive treatments is beneficial in nearly all cases of pyoderma (see Chapter 29)
- Nutritional support in the form of supplements or diets containing high levels of essential fatty acids and other cofactors may be beneficial

Review underlying cause, treatment plan and client compliance
Where chronic or recurrent pyoderma is secondary to persisting underlying cause, everything should be done to maximise the control of the underlying disease.

- A regular review of the status of the underlying disease
- Investigate possibility of new concomitant disease
- Regular review of treatment of underlying cause
- Regular review of flare factors
- Regular review of owner and patient compliance
  - Food trials and nutritional programmes of treatment
  - Drug administration
  - Shampooing and other labour intensive topical treatments
  - Avoidance of allergens and flare factors

Avoid the use of potentially immunosuppressive drugs during treatment

There are very few indications for the use of glucocorticoids or cyclosporin in pyoderma.

- Topical glucocorticoids may be beneficial in surface pyoderma
- Short courses of glucocorticoids may be beneficial in inflammatory lesions that have the potential to result in pyoderma
- Last resort in furunculosis
- Atopic patients maintained on these drugs who develop pyoderma

Otherwise glucocorticoids and cyclosporins are contraindicated during the treatment of pyoderma.

Progression of pyoderma

See Figure 27.1.

Appropriate aggressive treatment of pyoderma using the guidelines above should prevent the progression of pyoderma in most cases.

Surface pyoderma

- Most cases of surface pyoderma resolve in a few days as long as the underlying cause is addressed where it is likely to persist, e.g. skin fold pyoderma
- Mismanagement of surface pyoderma may however lead to superficial or deep pyoderma

Superficial pyoderma

- Superficial pyoderma is common in underlying inflammatory and endocrine dermatoses. The underlying cause should always be investigated and addressed, except where clinical signs are transient and resolve. However, in many cases the underlying condition is not adequately controlled in which case longer courses are indicated
- Management of these cases should be reviewed regularly and flare factors identified and treated
- Appropriate adjunctive and topical treatments will always be beneficial (see Chapter 29)
- Mismanagement of superficial pyoderma will lead to deep pyoderma

Deep pyoderma

- Deep pyoderma is a challenging condition to treat
- The underlying cause should always be identified and addressed
- Where the underlying cause is demodicosis, systemic antibiotic treatment should continue for several weeks beyond the cure of the primary condition
- Appropriate adjunctive and topical treatments are usually necessary (see Chapter 29)
- Mismanagement of deep pyoderma will lead to furunculosis

Furunculosis

- Furunculosis occurs frequently in demodicosis, callus pyoderma and in many other cases of deep pyoderma
- Progression to furunculosis should be avoided wherever possible by appropriate aggressive treatment of pyoderma

- Very long-term or sometimes permanent systemic antibiotic therapy may be needed in these cases as deep keratin will remain a nidus for infection as long as it is present
- Glucocorticoids should be avoided so that the foreign body reaction required to remove the keratin is not suppressed
- Appropriate adjunctive and topical treatment should be used
- The underlying cause should be addressed, although furunculosis is a self-perpetuating problem and even when the underlying cause is resolved the furunculosis will need further treatment
- Where all else fails the condition can be controlled by the use of anti-inflammatory treatments including glucocorticoids and cyclosporin long term, but this should be reserved for the last resort

Recurrent pyoderma

- The underlying cause should be addressed
- Adequately long courses of antibiotics
- Supportive and topical treatments
- Consider long-term low dose and pulse protocols for antibiotic use but controversial. Immunotherapy using commercial bacterial component products has been advocated

Resolution of pyoderma

Resolution of pyoderma is favoured by:

- Adequate appropriate early therapy
- Identify and address the underlying cause
- Good control of the underlying cause
- Avoid systemic glucocorticoids during treatment of all pyoderma
- Judicious and sparing use of topical glucocorticoids
- Good client and owner compliance

Progression of pyoderma

Progression of pyoderma is favoured by:

- Inappropriate antibiotic use
- Systemic glucocorticoid use
- Failure to identify and address underlying cause
- Poor control of underlying cause
- Flare factors
- Factors affecting immune and endocrine status of patient
- Inadequate use of antibiotics and supportive treatments

Bacterial overgrowth

This has recently been described:

- A surface overgrowth of bacteria, usually *Staphylococcus intermedius* which is poorly responsive to conventional treatment for pyoderma
- Underlying factors leading to overgrowth of bacterial flora should be identified and addressed

27.2.2 *MALASSEZIA* DERMATITIS AND OVERGROWTH

The management of *Malassezia* dermatitis is described in Chapter 11.3.

The primary treatment of *Malassezia* dermatitis is described in Chapter 26.2.

Malassezia dermatitis is an incompletely understood disease. The most common cause is a secondary complication of a primary underlying cause; hence the principles of treatment are similar to those of pyoderma. However, hypersensitivity reaction to *Malassezia* has been identified and allergen specific immunotherapy is a treatment option (Chapters 26.2.2 and 26.2.3).

The control of *Malassezia* dermatitis is important in increasing patient comfort whether it is the primary cause of the disease or a secondary flare factor.

Topical treatments
- Twice weekly bathing with 2% miconazole/2% chlorhexidine shampoo for a minim of 1 month. Long-term treatment is required if the underlying disease cannot be identified or addressed or if hypersensitivity to *Malassezia* has been identified
- Enilconazole 0.2% rinse in dogs only
- Enilconazole is toxic to cats

Supportive treatments
- *Malassezia* dermatitis responds to anti-inflammatory doses of systemic glucocorticoids. This may be caused by improvement of the underlying inflammatory disease. Glucocorticoids should not be used in the presence of demodicosis, dermatophytosis, other microbial disease or immunosuppressive or systemic disease

Outcome
- Always guarded due to either continuing presence of underlying cause or hypersensitivity to yeast. Long-term control frequently necessary

27.3 MANAGEMENT OF SCALING

Scaling is due to disruption of normal epidermal turnover and is frequently accompanied by increased greasiness. There are many underlying causes but management of scaling, especially in chronic skin disease, can increase patient comfort and cosmetic appearance considerably. The presence of dry skin and scale can significantly contribute to pruritus.

Except in mild or transient scaling, it is important to identify and address the underlying cause of scaling (see Chapter 5)

Primary treatments for scaling conditions are detailed in Chapter 26.

Secondary bacterial and yeast infections and overgrowth
Frequently secondary bacterial or yeast infection or overgrowth because of:
- Increased nutrients supplied by scale and grease
- Increased skin flora in inflammatory skin conditions

Treatment of Presenting Signs

Treatment of secondary pyoderma is detailed in Chapter 27.

Treatment of *Malassezia* dermatitis is detailed in Chapter 27.

27.3.1   SYSTEMIC TREATMENTS IN THE CONTROL OF SCALING

Several drugs have been shown to improve coat condition and reduce scaling and sebum production.

Essential fatty acids and cofactors   There are a number of compounds containing essential fatty acids combined with cofactors such as zinc, Vitamin E and Vitamin A available. Their main use is improving coat condition and scale.

Chinese herbal supplements   These are available as a nutritional supplement and may be of some benefit in the treatment of atopic dermatitis, but a considerable increase in coat condition has been seen with their use.

Nutritional supplements   These may improve scaling in some cases (see Chapter 27. 4).

Glucocorticoids   The risks of use may outweigh the benefits.

27.3.2   TOPICAL TREATMENTS IN THE CONTROL OF SCALING

Shampoos are beneficial in controlling scaling as they will remove skin debris and reduce the risk of secondary infection.

Ointments and creams are of less use.

The most gentle topical treatment which is effective should be used to avoid further disruption to normal epidermal turnover.

The specific actions of topical treatments in scaling disorders are detailed in Chapter 29.

27.4   NUTRITIONAL SUPPORT FOR DAMAGED SKIN

This can be supplied by:
• Food supplements
• Dermatological diet foods

These may be used in most dermatological diseases but may give most benefit in allergic skin disease.

Fatty acids
• Supplementation may improve the lipid barrier which is damaged in atopic dermatitis
• May favour production of non-inflammatory prostaglandins and leukotrienes

Treatment of Presenting Signs

Amino acids
• Precursors of collagen synthesis may be required in increased amounts in wound healing

Zinc
• Essential cofactor in collagen and protein synthesis, may be required in increased amounts in wound healing and immunological disease

Antioxidants
• Vitamin C and Vitamin E. Helps protect cells from the damaging effects of free radicals released from damaged tissue

Vitamin A
• Required for maintenance of epithelium. May be required in increased amounts in wound healing

Herbal supplementation
• A 3 herb chinese remedy based on a 20 herb human remedy has been launched as a nutritional supplement which may be beneficial in the treatment of atopic dermatitis

Reduced range of proteins, novel proteins and hydrolysed proteins
• These may be beneficial in reducing exposure to possible food antigens, but should not be confused with the much greater restriction which is necessary for a food elimination trial (Chapter 12). Of these diets only the lower molecular weight hydrolysed diets less than 13,000 kD are suitable for dietary trials and even these represent a compromise to the home cooked elimination diet.

Chapter 28

Use and Abuse of Glucocorticoids

28.1 INDICATIONS

The major indications for the use of glucocorticoids in dermatological conditions are listed in Table 28.1.

Glucocorticoid therapy should not be used:
• Long term in the absence of a diagnosis (Chapters 4 and 7)
• Long term in the presence of persistent clinical signs without exploring alternatives
• In any form of demodicosis
• In the presence of microbial disease

28.2 DOSE AND FORMULATION

28.2.1 PARENTERAL PRODUCTS

The only indication for parenteral use of glucocorticoids is in the short-term control of pruritus/inflammation in inappetant dogs or perioperatively. Short acting preparations should be used.

The only exception to this is for the long-term control of pruritus in cats where all efforts to pill have failed and other alternatives have been explored unsuccessfully.

Table 28.1   Indications for the use of glucocorticoids

Conditions where glucocorticoid therapy is indicated	Example
Short-term relief of pruritus where there are no contraindications	Hives, acute moist dermatitis Insect bite or sting
Control of pruritus as part of the treatment of ectoparasitic disease	Flea bite dermatitis, scabies
Treatment of diagnosed immune-mediated disease	Pemphigus foliaceus
Long-term treatment of diagnosed hypersensitivity dermatitis	Seasonal atopic dermatitis Otitis externa in atopic dermatitis
Palliation in neoplastic disease	Multicentric lymphoma Hepatocutaneous syndrome
Treatment in neoplastic disease	Epitheliotrophic lymphoma Mast cell tumour

28.2.2 ORAL SYSTEMIC PREPARATIONS

The only oral preparations which should be used are prednisolone or methylprednisolone tablets, or in some cases where available triamcinolone tablets.

28.2.3 TOPICAL CREAMS AND OINTMENTS

Topical creams and ointments are of limited use as they are licked off, although creams, ointments and sprays may be of use in localised lesions. Creams and ointments are particularly popular in human dermatology where the patient is less likely to lick the preparation off and therefore less likely to cause self-trauma, poisoning and worsening of lesions. There are many veterinary preparations available for topical use – the mildest treatments should be used first. If it considered necessary to use the stronger preparations this should only be done following a thorough review of diagnosis and treatment plan. The very potent human products should not be used.

28.2.4 DEXAMETHASONE SPRAYS

Dexamethasone sprays with limited absorption may be a useful adjunct in the treatment of more generalised disease on particularly severely affected areas, for example, inner pinnae, where tolerated by the patient.

28.2.5 SIDE-EFFECTS OF TOPICAL GLUCOCORTICOID USE

Although generally considered to be much safer than systemic glucocorticoids, topical products should be used only in the short term and with care. Side-effects include:

- Skin thinning
- Telangiectasia
- Hyperpigmentation
- Skin tearing
- Contact allergic dermatitis to vehicle or active ingredient

28.2.6 DOSE – SHORT-TERM USE

The commonly stated doses are listed below. However lower doses are often effective in mild inflammatory diseases. Aggressive initial treatment in more severe inflammatory and immune-mediated diseases is more likely to result in a resolution of signs or lower maintenance dose.

There is some individual variation in effective doses and a risk:benefit assessment should be made between efficacy and side-effects.

There is not a clear-cut distinction between anti-inflammatory and immunosuppressive doses.

Use and Abuse of Glucocorticoids

Gradual withdrawal of glucocorticoids is not necessary in dosing regimens of 2 weeks or less.

Glucocorticoids can be given at any time of day to domestic animals as naturally occurring cortisol levels show no set pattern.

Duration of action appears to be shorter in the smaller mammals, e.g. guinea pig.

Anti-inflammatory dose, dogs 1–2 mg/kg; cats 1–3 mg/kg; higher in small mammals.

Immunosuppressive dose, dogs 2–4 mg/kg; cats 3–6 mg/kg; higher in smaller mammals.

28.2.7 DOSE – LONG-TERM USE

There is no set maintenance dose for the long-term use of steroids. Every attempt should be used to ensure the lowest possible dose, which should be 0.5 mg/kg or preferably much less. This can be achieved by:

• Using a permanent dosing regime, rather than courses with interruptions
• Tapering the dose gradually – Chapter 28.3.1
• Use of steroid sparing measures
• Constant attention to control of flare factors
• Use of topical preparations, especially shampoos
• Constant review of diagnosis and treatment plans

Appendix 5: 'The safe use of steroids' is an example of an owner handout for use when prescribing long-term glucocorticoid therapy.

28.3 STEROID SPARING MEASURES

Although there is no safe dose of glucocorticoids, side-effects are dose dependent.

Steroid sparing measures should be adopted in all long-term glucocorticoid therapy.

28.3.1 TAPERING DOSE

The dose should be tapered gradually (no faster than a reduction every 2 weeks) to ensure that the lowest possible dose is achieved).

The dose should be reduced in small increments (no greater than 30% of dose) to achieve the lowest possible dose.

Introduce steroid sparing measures at the lowest possible tapered dose to achieve further reductions.

28.3.2 ALTERNATE DAY DOSING

It is recognised that alternate day dosing has less effect on the pituitary/hypophyseal/adrenal axis than daily dosing. It also usually results in a lower total maintenance dose of glucocorticoids.

Use and Abuse of Glucocorticoids

28.3.3 STEROID SPARING TREATMENTS

There are a number of ways of reducing the side-effects of glucocorticoids by reducing the dose even further.

In combination with other drugs (Chapters 27.1 and 27.4)
All of these uses are off label.
- Antihistamines have been reported to have a synergistic effect when used with glucocorticoids
- Cyclosporin has been used in combination with glucocorticoids to allow a considerable reduction in the doses, and hence side-effects, of both drugs
- Essential fatty acids have also been used to reduce the dose of glucocorticoids, though whether this is due to a primary effect on pruritus or due to improvement in coat condition and scaling is unknown
- Dog foods with high levels of essential fatty acids and cofactors have also been shown to offer some reduction in glucocorticoid use in some cases

Control of flare factors (Chapters 26.1, 27.1, 27.2 and 27.5)
All cases on long-term steroids should be monitored for secondary infections and ectoparasitic disease and treated for them to reduce pruritus. Dogs who develop demodicosis while on glucocorticoids should have the treatment withdrawn gradually and another antipruritic therapy identified.

Topical treatments (Chapter 29)
Ear cleaners and shampooing can reduce the dose of glucocorticoids used by:

- Removing debris and inflammatory products which may increase itch
- Reduce microbial load from the skin and ears
- Ameliorate the effects of increased humidity and temperature
- Reduce scaling and improving coat condition
- Antipruritic shampoos

28.4 SIDE-EFFECTS

Appendix 6 – 'Steroid side-effects' is an example of an owner handout for use when prescribing long-term glucocorticoid therapy which outlines the major side-effects seen with glucocorticoid use.

The most common side-effects associated with glucocorticoid use are listed in Table 28.2.

28.4.1 SHORT-TERM SIDE-EFFECTS

Some patients will not tolerate glucocorticoids at all, the most common side-effects being polydypsia and polyuria, leading to inappropriate urination. In these patients other means of therapy should be chosen or the diagnosis reviewed.

Table 28.2 Complications of systemic glucocorticoid use

Polydypsia, polyphagia, polyuria, inappropriate urination
Weight gain, muscle weakness, joint injury
Liver and metabolic disease
Iatrogenic HAC
Depression, behaviour changes
Demodicosis
Pyoderma, dermatophytosis
Cystitis
Gastric ulceration
Hairloss, scaling, skin thinning

Complications of long-term glucocorticoid use

- Some dogs can be maintained on glucocorticoids for many years without visible side-effects
- However, these patients should be carefully monitored and their weight restricted. Larger dogs may become susceptible to joint injury as a result of weight gain and tendon and ligament weakening
- It is important not to mistake iatrogenic HAC, pyoderma and demodicosis for a worsening in the inflammatory condition. Review of diagnosis, including mandatory skin scrapings should always be undertaken before increasing the dose of glucocorticoids or if the condition worsens

28.5 CONTRAINDICATIONS

The main contraindications for glucocorticoids are listed in Table 28.3.

Table 28.3 Contraindications for the use of glucocorticoids

Conditions where glucocorticoids are contraindicated	Example
Ectoparasitic disease where the immune system is compromised	Demodicosis Feline scabies associated with systemic disease
Microbial disease	Dermatophytosis Other fungal infections Pyoderma
Systemic disease	Liver disease
Endocrine disease affecting cortisol metabolism	Calcinosis cutis in HAC Diabetic dermatosis
Presence of side-effects	Inappropriate urination Weight gain Pancreatitis
Concomitant NSAIDs	Concomitant degenerative joint disease and hypersensitivity dermatitis
Concomitant antibiotics	Skin infections Systemic infections

Although contraindicated in most microbial disease there is often a good response to glucocorticoids in *Malassezia* dermatitis. This may be a primary effect or due to the improvement of underlying inflammatory disease.

Although glucocorticoids are contraindicated in liver disease, they may be used with some success in the palliative treatment of superficial necrolytic dermatitis (hepatocutaneous syndrome, metabolic epidermal necrosis, necrolytic migratory erythema).

The injudicious use of glucocorticoids in pyoderma is often responsible for the progression of pyoderma (Chapter 27.2).

Chapter 29

Topical Treatments

Topical treatments are nearly always beneficial in the treatment of skin disease but because of poor owner and patient compliance they are frequently underused. The reasons for poor owner compliance are well justified. Table 29.1 demonstrates why this is often the case, time taken to apply topical treatments and unrealistic expectations being the most important, closely followed by poor patient compliance (especially in cats).

29.1 USE OF TOPICAL PREPARATIONS

Treat the primary disease
- Sprays, washes, rinses, spot-ons and line-ons for ectoparasitic disease and fungal infections
- Antimicrobial shampoos for superficial pyoderma, *Malassezia* dermatitis and dermatophytosis

Sole method of treatment
- Inflammatory lesions
- Antimicrobial shampoos in acute superficial pyoderma
- Creams, ointments and sprays in acute moist dermatitis
- Keratolytic/keratoplastic shampoos in mild scaling dermatoses

Treat secondary complications and flare factors
- Shampoos used to control scaling, pyoderma and secondary *Malassezia* dermatitis
- Antipruritic sprays and ointments
  - Steroid sprays in atopic dermatitis
  - Antipruritic ointments

Adjunctive treatments
- Miconazole shampoos in dermatophytosis
- Topical antibacterials in superficial and deep pyoderma
- Antimicrobial shampoos in generalised demodicosis
- Nearly all patients suffering from any dermatosis will benefit from some form of topical treatment, as long as the appropriate treatment is used in the correct way
- Normal skin may also benefit from shampooing
  - Shampooing removes grease, debris and scale from coats
  - Deodorising shampoos and sprays
  - Conditioning shampoos and sprays

Topical treatments are frequently underused, partly because, with so many new drugs available to treat the primary disease, it is easy to forget that a topical treatment is a useful aid to treatment. Many clinicians have also experienced a poor response to treatment with topical treatments due to poor choice of product, unrealistic expectations for efficacy and poor owner and patient compliance.

29.2 INAPPROPRIATE USE OF TOPICAL PRODUCTS CAN BE HARMFUL

- Steroid containing compounds should be avoided in:
  - Deep pyoderma
  - Dermatophytosis
  - Demodicosis
- Bleaching and astringent shampoos, and those containing tar and sulphur should be used with caution
- Shampoos should be rinsed thoroughly to avoid local irritant reactions

29.3 FORMULATIONS OF TOPICAL TREATMENTS

- Shampoos
- Creams and ointments
- Washes and rinses
- Sprays, spot-ons and line-ons
- Aural preparations

29.3.1 SHAMPOOS

Benefits of shampooing
- Safe method of delivering active ingredients to the skin reducing the need for, and duration of, systemic therapy
  - In primary disease, such as dermatophytosis, juvenile impetigo
  - In secondary disease such as pyoderma
  - Antipruritic shampoo used as a steroid sparing measure
- Remove scale, bacteria, yeasts, debris and inflammatory products from the skin
  - Increases patient comfort
  - Physically removes irritant agents
  - Physically removes allergens from skin surface
  - Reduces bacterial and yeast contamination of skin surface, hence reducing secondary infections
  - Improves coat condition, appearance and smell, improving owner tolerance

Correct use of shampoos is vital. Shampoos are frequently used incorrectly, often because of poor patient compliance, but insufficient contact time renders the product useless and insufficient rinsing can result in irritant reactions and surface pyoderma, especially intertrigo.

Table 29.1 outlines the important factors in choosing and using a shampoo.

Topical Treatments

Table 29.1 Maximising beneficial effects of topical treatments

Choice of product	Avoid using astringent, bleaching or irritant treatments where possible Use the gentlest product first Glucocorticoids contraindicated in demodicosis, dermatophytosis, pyoderma
Use of product	Clip hair where necessary Adequate contact time with skin Thorough rinsing where appropriate Correct frequency for product
Owner compliance	Essential Many topical products are time consuming Precise instructions followed for success
Client expectations	Useful adjuncts, rarely sufficient on their own Long-term use required for control rather than cure Slow onset of improvement often seen
Address underlying causes	Frequent cause of client dissatisfaction is lack of cure

Use veterinary products
- The pH of canine skin is a neutral 7 compared with the acidic 5.5 of humans. Use of human shampoos may produce irritant reactions
- Additives to human shampoos – perfumes, etc., may produce irritant reactions and contact sensitisation
- Toxic effects may be seen when human products are licked off by the patient as ingestion is less of a consideration in humans
- Some herbal shampoos are toxic when ingested

Active ingredients in shampoos
- The common active ingredients in shampoos are listed in Table 29.2

Emollients and moisturisers
- Improve coat condition
- Reduce water loss from skin
- Keratoplastic
- Present in many shampoos for normal skin
- Useful in mild scaling dermatoses
- Used in rinses to improve coat condition and aid grooming

Antiparasitic shampoos
- These have largely fallen into disuse.
- Less effective than rinses, sprays, spot-ons, collars, etc., as they are rinsed off and lack residual effect
- Used for rapid 'knock-down' effect
- Remove scale, debris, exudate and oil which is beneficial in reducing pruritus
- Physically remove parasites, larvae and eggs, speeding response to treatment
- Should not be used with other ectoparasiticides due to cumulative toxic effects
- Most contain synthetic pyrethroids or selenium sulphide

Table 29.2 Active ingredients in shampoos and their uses

Shampoo	Active ingredient	Indication
Emollients and moisturisers (keratoplastic)	Present in many shampoos Colloidal oatmeal Fatty acids Urea Chitosanide Glycerine	Mild scaling Dry skin and hair coat Normal skin Erythema Hypersensitivity dermatitis
Antimicrobial fungal/yeast shampoos	Chlorhexidine Miconazole/chlorhexidine Povidone iodine Selenium sulphide	Secondary pyoderma Dermatophytosis/yeast infections Excess grease and scale
Antiseptic shampoos	Benzoyl peroxide Ethyl oxide Chlorhexidine Piroctone olamine Tea tree oil	Superficial secondary pyoderma, e.g. hypothyroidism, HAC and diabetes mellitus Demodicosis Hypersensitivity dermatitis
Antiseborrhoeic shampoos (keratoplastic and keratolytic)	Shampoos containing sulphur, tar, selenium sulphide, salicylic acid Linoleic acid Gamma linolenic acid	Excess scale and grease Primary scaling disorders Secondary scaling disorders Hypersensitivity dermatitis
Moderation of sebum production	Vitamin B6 Zinc gluconate	Primary and secondary scaling disorders
Antipruritic	Monosaccharides Vitamin E Salicylic acid Sulphur	Pruritic skin disease with minimal secondary change

Antifungal/anti-yeast shampoos
- *Malassezia* dermatitis can be treated using twice weekly miconazole/chlorhexidine shampoos
- Miconazole/chlorhexidine shampoos can be used in the treatment of *Malassezia* dermatitis and dermatophytosis
- More stubborn cases requiring systemic therapy benefit from use of miconazole/chlorhexidine shampoos as an adjunct
- Topical treatment useful in reducing transmission between animals in dermatophytosis

Antibacterial shampoos
- Used as the sole treatment in some mild surface and superficial pyoderma
  - Acute moist dermatitis
  - Intertrigo
  - Juvenile impetigo
  - Mild superficial pyoderma
- Used as an adjunctive treatment in secondary pyodermas
  - Parasitic dermatitis
  - Hypersensitivity dermatitis

Topical Treatments

- Other immune-mediated disease
- Endocrine disease
- Essential in the treatment of demodicosis
- Keratolytic and comedolytic effect of benzoyl peroxide shampoos can be beneficial in superficial and deep pyoderma
- 'Follicle flushing' effect of benzoyl peroxide is now considered to be controversial
- In less severe dermatoses use milder shampoos first to avoid irritant reactions and exacerbation of signs
  - Ethyl lactate is the least likely to produce an irritant reaction; chlorhexidine, miconazole and benzoyl peroxide have the greatest antibacterial effect

Keratinoplastic and keratinolytic shampoos (shampoos for seborrhoeic conditions)
- Active ingredients include tar, sulphur, selenium sulphide, salicylic acid, alone or in combination
- Used in either primary or secondary keratinisation defects as sole treatment or useful adjunct
- Nearly all seborrhoeic patients benefit greatly from their use whether the keratinisation defect is primary or secondary
- Remove excess grease and scale (keratolytic)
- Increase epidermal cell turnover time and promote normal keratinocyte and sebaceous gland function (keratoplastic)
- Cleansing and reduce smell
- Reduce surface bacterial and yeast population
- Can be irritant, especially if tar is in high concentration
- Tar and sulphur now being superceded

Antipruritic shampoos
- All shampoos used correctly have some antipruritic effect as they physically remove grease, scale and bacteria
- Some shampoos specifically contain antipruritic agents such as colloidal oatmeal and essential fatty acids, sulphur and salicylic acid
- Some moisturisers have some direct antipruritic action
- Usually used as an adjunct to systemic treatment except in mild cases
- There are some effective glucocorticoid and tacrolimus containing topical compounds, but not as yet veterinary licensed

Choice of shampoo
Often complex.

- The correct shampoo may be too irritant for the patient, especially where there is broken or inflamed skin
- Use the gentlest appropriate treatment first
- Be aware of sensitising reactions
- Test small areas of skin before shampooing the body
- Alternating shampoos can be useful if
  - The effective shampoo is too irritant to use every time

- There is a complex problem, e.g. pyoderma combined with inflammation and pruritus
- Spray and lotion formulations can be used to prolong intervals between shampooing where this is desirable, but be aware of build up on the skin

29.3.2 CREAMS AND OINTMENTS

Use of creams and ointments
- Sole treatment of localised lesions such as acute moist dermatitis, acral lick dermatitis, minor wounds and abrasions
- Antipruritic ointments, glucocorticoids and other compounds
- Emollients
- Antibacterial
- Frequently polypharmaceutical and imprecise action
- To treat secondary complications of underlying disease – surface and superficial pyoderma, excoriations due to self-trauma
- As an adjunct to systemic therapy as in folliculitis where areas such as the chin and muzzle need specific attention

Limitations and complications associated with the use of creams and ointments
- Licking of topical product
  - Reduces contact time
  - Increased self-trauma
- Messy to use
  - Handling considerations for owners, including contact sensitisation
  - Build of skin debris leading to loss of efficacy
- Systemic absorption of creams and ointments can be underestimated
- Some steroid containing preparations have measurable effects on adrenal/pituitary/hypothalamic axis
- Most are antibiotic/steroid combinations which should not be used for:
  - Pyoderma
  - Dermatophytosis
  - Demodicosis
- Undesirable reactions
  - Irritant
  - Idiosyncratic
  - Some active ingredients are recognised contact sensitisers

29.3.3 WASHES AND RINSES

Use of washes and rinses
- Sole treatment of primary condition
  - Enilconazole in the treatment of dermatophytosis in dogs and small mammals (toxic to cats)
  - Amitraz in the primary treatment of demodicosis

- Secondary adjunctive treatment
  ○ Enilconazole in the treatment of dermatophytosis as above
- Conditioning washes and rinses as an aid to grooming in normal dogs
- Emollients in scaling dermatoses

Limitations of washes and rinses
- Rinsed off by shampooing and swimming
- Skin contact restricted by hair coat
- Toxicity of enilconazole in cats
- Irritant reactions

29.3.4 SPRAYS, SPOT-ONS AND LINE-ONS

Most of these products are formulated for the primary control of ectoparasitic conditions (see Chapter 26).

Glucocorticoid sprays in the control of pruritus. A veterinary licensed glucocorticoid spray has been formulated with a data sheet claim for minimal systemic absorption at the recommended rates of spraying.

29.3.5 AURAL PREPARATIONS

Chapter 20 describes the management of aural disease.

Use of topical aural preparations
The main advantages and disadvantages of topical aural preparations are shown in Table 29.3.

Treatment of primary ear disease
- Topical acaricidal preparations for ectoparasitic treatment

Ear washes for the control of factors exacerbating ear disease
- Wax accumulation
- Humidity due to conformational and environmental factors
- Control of secondary complications of primary aural disease
- Flushing and removal of wax, debris and irritant products of infection and inflammation

Antibiotic and glucocorticoid preparations
- Occasional judicious use in the control of secondary bacterial and yeast infections where the primary cause has been identified and addressed
- Short-term use for the control of secondary infection and inflammation where the primary cause is transient and is readily resolved, e.g. otocariasis, foreign body (after removal), swimming or grooming incident

Topical Treatments

Table 29.3 Advantages and disadvantages of topical aural preparations

Advantages	Disadvantages
Usually well tolerated by patient	May be difficult to use in painful ears
Good contact achieved at site of infection/inflammation	May be messy and cause hair matting and maceration of tissues
Most modern topical preparations very effective at treating secondary bacterial infections and inflammation	Underlying cause is not usually addressed and may go unidentified
Rapid onset of action	May obscure underlying cause, e.g. foreign body
Will reduce clinical signs and increase patient comfort in chronic otitis	Will not halt progression of primary ear disease and change to ear canal
Local treatment reduces systemic effects of glucocorticoid use	Many topical glucocorticoid preparations are absorbed sufficiently to demonstrate effects on hypophyseal/pituitary/adrenal axis
	Many cannot be used where the tympanic membrane is ruptured

Abuse of topical aural preparatons

In cases of chronic or recurrent aural disease the underlying cause should be identified and addressed.

Long-term use of topical aural preparations will not halt the progression of chronic or recurrent aural disease.

Changing the type of topical aural preparation used is unlikely to improve the outcome.

Long-term empirical use of polypharmaceutical topical aural preparations favour growth of resistant bacteria in the ear in an ideal environment to culture them, especially *Pseudomonas* spp.

Use of ear wicks

Ear wicks have been used with some success in chronic recurrent otitis externa where secondary bacterial infection and inflammation are significant.

1 Examine the ear under general anaesthesia
2 Take samples for cytological examination for identification of bacteria
3 Take bacteriological swabs for microbial culture
4 Clean the ear thoroughly
5 Use a drying preparation, such as weak boric acid solution
6 Place the ear wick at the junction of the vertical and horizontal canal with the aid of an auroscope
7 Add 1 ml triz EDTA and 1 ml of appropriate antibiotic based on cytological examination or preferably culture and sensitivity testing
8 Add 1 ml steroid solution where appropriate
9 Add further solution after 2–3 days
10 Remove the ear wicks under sedation or general anaesthetic after 4–5 days and repeat the process if necessary
11 Reassess the underlying cause of the otitis externa

Topical Treatments

Use of ear cleaners

Ear cleaners are valuable in ear disease whatever the cause.

- Antiseptic – promote a slightly acidic environment, discouraging microbial growth
- Flushing – removal of cerumen and debris from the ear canal towards the outside
- Drying – discouraging microbial growth

Ear cleaners should be used constantly in chronic/recurrent otitis externa or dogs or cats predisposed to otitis externa. The flushing and antibacterial effects of the ear cleaners on the market are currently under investigation.

Treatment of chronic and recurrent otitis externa

The management of chronic/recurrent otitis externa is described in Chapter 20.

- Investigate the underlying cause – the most common is hypersensitivity dermatitis
- The best way to treat bacterial otitis externa is to prevent the occurrence of predisposing factors
- Use ear cleaners aggressively to improve the environment in the ear canal
- Use antibiotic and glucocorticoid preparations with caution and with a regular review of the diagnosis and underlying causes

APPENDICES

Appendix 1

History Form

HISTORY FORM

Owner's complaint

GENERAL HISTORY

Environment and lifestyle

Breed		Sex		Age	
Date wormed		Date vaccinated		Neutered/Entire	
Age acquired			General diet		
Other dogs		Other animals		Owners affected	
Other pet contact		Wildlife/livestock contact		Travel history	

Previous medical history (excluding skin diseases)

Condition	Dates	Treatments given	Response

Current Health

General Demeanour	Exercise Tolerance
Appetite Normal / Poor / Excessive / Increasing	Thirst Normal / Poor / Excessive / Increasing
Weight Thin / Fair / Good / Fat / Obese	Decreasing / Increasing / Stable
GI signs	Respiratory signs
Cardiovascular signs	Musculoskeletal signs
Neurological signs	Other

Tests performed

Test	Result

DERMATOLOGICAL HISTORY

General dermatological history

Age at onset	First signs
Severity of condition 1 2 3 4 5	Intermittent / Persistent
Improving/Stable/Fluctuating/Worsening	

Response to treatments, diets, supplements
0 = none, 2 = 20% 3 = 50%, 4 = 80%, 5 = 100%

Treatment	Names	Dates	% response	Duration of action
Drugs				
Diets				
Supplements				
Ectoparasiticides				
Other				

Owner patient score
0 = absent, 1 = mild 2 = moderate 3 = severe

	At onset	Current	Previous	Comments, triggers and spread
Itch				
Hairloss				
Smell				
Total area affected				
Spots				
Scaling and crusting				
Face				
Legs and feet				
Dorsum				
Ventrum				
Ears				

Environmental history

General Rural / Coastal / Urban / Suburban	
Daytime Inside / Outside / Car Free access / Restricted (give area)	
Nighttime Inside / Outside Upstairs / Downstairs Own bed / Owner's bed	
Bedding	**Cleaning of bedding**
Other	

Appendix 2
Clinical Examination

CLINICAL EXAMINATION

General Examination

Eyes, ears, nose, mouth	Musculoskeletal system
Cardiovascular/Respiratory systems	GI system
Neurological signs	Other observations e.g. lymphadenopathy

Dermatological Examination

Hairloss 0 1 2 3	Erythema 0 1 2 3
Hyperpigmentation 0 1 2 3	Thickening and lichenification 0 1 2 3
Scale 0 1 2 3	Excoriation 0 1 2 3
Greasiness 0 1 2 3	Sweating 0 1 2 3

Description of lesions (see Chapter 2)

Nodules, plaques and masses	Macules/Papules/Pustules/Vesicles
Change in pigmentation	

Areas affected

Face 0 1 2 3	Ears 0 1 2 3
Periorbital skin 0 1 2 3	Axillae and groin 0 1 2 3
Feet 0 1 2 3	Legs 0 1 2 3
Dorsum 0 1 2 3	Ventrum 0 1 2 3

Areas spared

Brief summary

Action plan

Appendix 3
Testing Food Intolerance
Owner Handout

We tend to refer to these as food allergies, but other types of skin adverse reaction to food can also occur, all of which can lead to your dog or cat becoming itchy. There are a few facts that can help when investigating a possible reaction to diet. It is always worth food trialling as, if this is the cause, we have the ideal treatment – controlling an allergic reaction without the use of drugs.

1 **How common is food intolerance?** Opinions vary, but food intolerance may account for between 5% and 25% of itchy dogs. It is likely that many dogs remain undiagnosed as it is difficult and time consuming to test for food reactions.

2 **Is there a simple test for food intolerance?** There is a blood test available for testing for food reactions, but although it may help us to choose the foods for a food trial, or can give an idea as to whether your pet may be predisposed to food intolerance, we cannot as yet rely on the test alone for the diagnosis of food reactions, so the only reliable way to test for food intolerance is to put the pet on a very restricted diet for 6–12 weeks. It is not possible to rule out food intolerance on the results of a blood test alone.

3 **What should I feed my dog when on a food trial?** The 'gold standard' diet is a home-cooked protein which they are not usually fed (usually a specific type of meat/fish), combined with a single carbohydrate which they are not usually fed (e.g. rice or potato). With the wide variety of pet foods available today, this is getting increasingly difficult. You should only start a food trial following a full discussion with your veterinary surgeon.

4 **What should I feed my cat on a food trial?** Feed only a specific type of home-cooked protein (meat or fish), as they will not usually eat a dull carbohydrate.

5 **Can any pet be food trialled?** Pets under 12–18 months of age cannot be food trialled on home-cooked diets. Healthy adult pets can cope with this dietary imbalance for 6–12 weeks but they should not be fed this food long term as it doesn't contain everything that your pet needs to maintain good health. Again it is vital that you discuss this with your veterinary surgeon before starting a food trial.

6 **Can I add anything to the diet to make it more palatable?** No, food trialling has to be strict. If this is not possible, a commercial hydrolysed diet may be the answer. Your pet may lose weight and start scavenging on the restricted diet but they will soon recover when the trial is over. There is no point in starting a food trial if you don't think you can be strict enough for long enough.

7 **My cat goes out, can I still do a food trial?** As long as you accept the compromise that he may 'eat out' especially if what he is offered at home is boring, it is still worthwhile. Although less likely to work, it is still most likely to be something that you are feeding that he is reacting to, so you may still get a valid response.

8 **Will a change of brand of food help?** No, most petfoods are composed of the same protein and carbohydrate groups due to price and availability of foodstuffs globally,

so it would be very unlikely that you would find a brand that gave an improvement in his skin condition. Many people find this out the hard way – some have tried 10 or 15 brands of pet food before asking for professional advice.

9 **Can I use one of the hypoallergenic brands on the market?** These diets are not usually restricted enough for food trialling although they will almost certainly be useful in finding a diet which your pet can eat once the diagnosis has been made. Trace ingredients added to produce a balanced diet may cause your pet not to respond to the food trial.

10 **It is too difficult to do a home-cooked trial, can I still do a food trial?** There are now hydrolysed diets on the market. The theory is that these diets are of very low molecular weight and so cannot trigger an allergic reaction. These diets, which come in tinned and dried forms, can be used successfully in most cases although a small number will fail to respond. So many people have busy lives these days that these are becoming the most common way of food trialling pets. It is better to succeed with a hydrolysed diet than fail with a home-cooked diet.

Rules of the food trial

Food trialling is a very helpful diagnostic procedure in finding out the cause of your pet's itch, but is very time consuming and challenging.

The exact choice of food will be discussed with you depending on your pet's existing diet and lifestyle.

1 The pet must not eat any other food at any time.
2 Even one cheat a week will make the trial invalid.
3 No treats or chews during the trial.
4 All pets in the same house should be fed the same or kept strictly apart during eating opportunities.
5 Clear up all food scraps straight away and feed the cat up high.
6 Make sure the bins and compost heaps are secure.
7 Make sure everyone in the household, your friends and neighbours know that your pet is on a restricted diet.
8 It is very hard to food trial pets in houses where there are very young children or very old people.
9 Don't try to food trial during celebrations, for example, Christmas – there is too much interesting food around in unrestricted places.
10 Nothing can be added to the trial diet. Home-cooked diets can be boiled or dry roasted, but no additions, even seasonings can be made.
11 No fast food or pet packs can be used – original raw ingredients only and potatoes should be peeled as the skins may contain contaminants.
12 We can use treatments to control your pet's symptoms in a very controlled way during the trial. You will need to discuss this with your vet as the trial progresses.

We know how difficult this is – it is not always possible to do this for 6–12 weeks. It is better to be realistic and not start a food trial than to struggle with something which is impossible in your household.

Ring in every 3 weeks when on a food trial for advice on how to keep your pet comfortable and how to make it to the finish. We will also give you a bit of encouragement.

Appendix 4

Advice on the Use of Medicinal Products

While every effort has been made to give accurate doses for the drugs used in treatments in this book, the veterinary surgeon should follow the current recommendations of the data sheet for any licensed products and the most up to date texts and literature for any product used off label.

There are some conditions in veterinary dermatology for which there is no licensed drug or for which, due to the chronicity of the conditions, drugs may need to be used in a manner other than that which is described on the data sheet accompanying the product. It should be borne in mind that, while all drugs have the potential to produce adverse effects or may not be 100% efficacious, some of the drugs that we use are toxic to both our patients and their owners, as well as the environment.

There are strict regulations on the use of medicinal products in animals governed by administrative bodies in all countries, for example, the Veterinary Medicines Directorate in the UK and the Food and Drugs Administration in the USA.

There are many drugs with veterinary licences and data sheets which outline the use of these drugs. Wherever there is a suitable veterinary licensed product for a condition, this should be used according to the data sheet recommendations. Whenever it is unavoidable to use a product in an off label manner or a product licensed for another species, or an imported product, the regulations and guidelines of the relevant government should be followed. For example, the Cascade gives guidance from the Veterinary Medicines Directorate on the use of medicinal products in the UK.

Further information can be found on the following websites:
For the UK, www.vmd.gov.uk
For the USA, www.fda.gov
For Australia, www.avpma.gov.au
For Europe, www.emea.europa.eu

Consideration should always be given to the impact on human health and the environment when using veterinary medicinal products as well as adverse reactions and the risk of handling to owners when administering the products.

Adverse reactions
- Owners should be advised of the risk of adverse reaction to all drugs
- The data sheet should be given to the owner where possible so that there is evidence that this obligation has been fulfilled
- The attention of the owner should be especially drawn to specific adverse reactions and those which may affect anyone handling the patient
- Adverse reactions should be reported to the relevant authority

Handling veterinary medicines

- The owner should be advised to use gloves when using all veterinary medicinal products. This is especially important when handling topical products, or drugs to which the owner may become sensitised or where toxicity can be an issue
- Drugs should be dispensed in child proof containers and be stored where children and animals cannot gain access
- Drugs for animals should not be stored in the same cupboard as drugs for humans
- Pill splitting should be avoided. Where this is necessary, a pill splitting device should be supplied
- Where pill splitting is contraindicated less frequent dosing of the whole pill should be considered, or consider another formulation
- Home made formulations should be avoided
- Owners should be advised where possible sensitisations may occur. The most common of these is penicillins

Disposal of veterinary medicines

- All veterinary medicines should be disposed of in accordance with the pharmaceutical waste regulations of the appropriate country
- Particular care should be taken to ensure that no medicines enter water courses where they may damage the environment
- Be aware that especially ectoparasiticides can be very toxic

Appendix 5

Safe Use of Glucocorticoids

Owner Handout

The title is a bit misleading as there is no such thing as a completely safe dose of glucocorticoids. All drugs and herbal remedies have the potential to produce side-effects and adverse effects. However, in some cases, they are the only effective form of treatment and they can be used safely by following a few rules combined with carefully monitoring the patients' progress.

A short course of steroids to treat an inflammatory condition causing discomfort is unlikely to cause problems.

- Effectively control the discomfort of an insect sting or sudden allergic reaction
- Sudden cases of irritation or rash where they only need to be used for a short time
- Pets with seasonal allergies (e.g. grass and tree pollens) are often best treated with a course of steroids until the itch settles down
- To ease patient's discomfort when they are being treated for other known conditions such as fleas or other parasites

Long-term steroid treatment should only be considered if we know the condition we are treating and other forms of treatment are not available to you, or your pet does not tolerate them, or if other forms of treatment turn out to not be effective.

- Steroids are most commonly used in the treatment of allergy. It is important where possible to confirm that the problem is due to allergic reaction before using steroids long term as they can mask other causes of disease. Tests can be done to find out exactly what the problem is before opting for long-term steroid use. Even in cases of allergy there are other forms of treatment available and other drugs which can be used. None are more effective than steroids, but some are much safer.

Long-term steroid treatment should only be given in tablet form (prednisolone or medrone tablets given daily or every other day). Historically pets have been given long-acting injections to control their itch. We now know that this is not a good idea.

- The injections do not control the problem as effectively as daily tablets because the dose is inconsistent – high when the drug is first given, low later on. This results in higher doses being given than when tablets are used
- Daily tablets are safer. If there are side-effects, they can be stopped immediately and side-effects stop rapidly. Once the injection is given it cannot be removed. Again because the tablets work better smaller, safer doses are given
- It is recognised that steroids are safer if they are given every other day, so that the body has 'a day off' from treatment. This is not possible with injections

We know that daily pill-giving is not easy.

However, with perseverance and bribery it is usually possible and, after a bumpy 2–3 weeks at the start of treatment, even the most awkward cat will usually cooperate. We also have aids to help in giving tablets and show you the best way to achieve success.

Steroid treatment should not be given to pets suffering from certain conditions or on certain other treatments.

Check with your vet if you are not sure if your pet is completely well otherwise or if he/she is on any other treatment. Circumstances where you probably will not be able to give steroids include:
- If your pet has any bacterial, fungal or viral disease (infection)
- If your pet is on any NSAID (non-steroidal drug, commonly used for arthritis)
- If your pet is on antibiotics
- If your pet has a disease affecting the immune system
- If your pet has diabetes or another condition known as Cushing's syndrome (HAC)

Long-term steroid treatment should be tailored to each individual patient.

In the main it is safer to give steroids at a high dose initially, then gradually reduce the dose to a level where they are comfortable with only very minor side-effects, than to give occasional courses of higher dose steroids, but this needs to be worked out for each patient and so your pet will need close monitoring, especially in the early stages of treatment.

There are many things which can be done to reduce the dose of steroids which your pet needs.

Other less effective drugs can be used at the same time as steroids to reduce the dose that your pet needs to be given. While rarely enough to control the problem by themselves, they can significantly reduce the dose of steroids given. These drugs include antihistamines, essential fatty acids and other herbal-type products, but please ask the vet about this rather than experimenting on your own, as there are certain drugs which can be dangerous when used in combination with steroids.

Shampooing will almost always help an inflamed skin. But remember always to ask your vet about this rather than try pet shop and health shop remedies. Remember that products bought for humans are often not suitable for dogs and cats. Shampooing cats can be very difficult.

Appendix 6

Side-Effects Seen When Steroids are Given

Owner Handout

1. If you see any of the following DO NOT stop the tablets without consulting the vet. Stopping the treatment abruptly may cause further health problems, especially when steroids have been given at high doses or for a long time.
2. We do not see osteoporosis as experienced by humans on long term steroid therapy very often.
3. All patients vary in the type and severity of side-effects they show. Some patients tolerate quite high doses while some show serious side-effects even on very low doses. In the main, cats show fewer side-effects on steroids than dogs and tolerate higher doses, but everyone has an individual response.
4. Most steroid side-effects are reversible – that is they will get better when your pet stops taking the drugs.

What you may see	Consequences	What you should do
Increased thirst *Common*	Loss of house training, incontinence	Consult the vet if you experience problems, consult the vet if thirst persists on long-term usage
Increased appetite *Common*	Weight gain, bin raiding and lethargy	Don't feed more. If problems are severe, consult the vet. Monitor weight and report increase to vet. If your pet is bin-raiding and scavenging, consult the vet urgently as this is dangerous (they may eat something they shouldn't)
Dullness depression *Uncommon*	Unhappy pet, dogs unwilling to go for walks, very occasionally aggression	Consult the vet, although it may pass after a couple of days on the tablets, but treatment will have to be discontinued if it persists
Pot-bellied, unfit appearance, weight loss, muscle wastage *Uncommon, but warning sign of more serious problem*	May be associated with increase in thirst and appetite, coughing	Do not stop giving the tablets until you have consulted the vet. It is likely that another form of treatment will have to be given and the problem will resolve naturally

(Continued)

(Continued)

Side-Effects Seen When Steroids are Given

What you may see	Consequences	What you should do
Weak muscles, ligaments and tendons *Common in long-term treatment, especially if high dose*	Weakened ligaments and tendons will be more prone to injury, especially if there is already weight gain. This is most important in big dogs	Report your concerns to the vet at the next re-examination
Scaly thin, spotty skin infections, hair loss *Common*	Hairloss is commonly seen in long-term steroid use, but unhealthy looking skin may be a warning sign of more serious side-effects	Consult your vet. Shampooing and essential fatty acids can help treat the scaly skin commonly seen in dogs on long-term steroids
Sudden increase in thirst when previously stable *Uncommon*	May be an early warning sign of uncommon but serious side-effects such as Cushing's syndrome, liver disease, pancreatic disease	Consult your vet with a urine sample if possible
Inappetance or not eating at all *Very uncommon*	May be an early warning sign of uncommon but serious side-effects such as Cushing's syndrome, liver disease, pancreatic disease. Also possibly an infection	Consult your vet straight away
Vomiting *Very uncommon*	May be due to gastric irritation or ulceration which can occur on long-term steroid therapy, especially high dose, infection or Cushing's liver or pancreatic disease	Consult your vet straight away
Blood in the urine *Very uncommon*	May be cystitis (pets on steroids are more susceptible)	Consult your vet with a urine sample if possible
Blood in the faeces or dark faeces (motions, stools) *Very uncommon*	May be due to gastric or bowel irritation or ulceration	Consult your vet straight away
Sudden or persistent worsening of skin irritation, infections, hair loss, smell, etc. *Very uncommon*	May be due to infections which are more likely in pets on steroids such as mite infestation and ringworm, or Cushing's disease which can be a side-effect of long-term usage or could be skin problem getting worse	Consult your vet straight away

This list does not contain all the problems, so if you are worried about any aspect of your pet's health, you should consult your veterinary surgeon.

INDEX